Praise for *Run Li...*

"We all have a million excuses to skip a daily run, but you only need 365 antidotes to change your life. And here they are, all funny, wise, and warm. Lace up, girls!"
—Kathrine Switzer, founder 261 Fearless,
and author of *Marathon Woman*

"*Run Like a Girl 365 Days a Year* motivates, inspires, and celebrates what it means to be a female athlete. It reminds and prepares us to be the best version of ourselves."
—Christie Pearce Rampone, former captain of the US women's
National soccer team and three-time Olympic gold medalist

"Mina Samuels's *Run Like a Girl 365 Days a Year* speaks to the inner athlete in all of us. Both inspirational and practical, this book is a great companion on your athletic journey. Offering bite-sized prompts for thought and action, readers will learn, and laugh, and grow."
—Samantha J. Brennan, co-founder of Fit Is a Feminist Issue
and co-author of *Fit at Mid-Life: A Feminist Fitness Journey*

"As an expressive boy full of joy, my older brother tried to stifle my light. He bullied me by calling me a sissy and saying, 'you run like a girl.' In life, hidden in the forces that pull us down is the energy to lift us up. In retaliation, I learned to flip and fly, moving faster than anyone around me. Mina brings new meaning to that phrase with her insightful and masterful book *Run Like a Girl 365 Days a Year*. Her physical, mental, and spiritual journey align with both truth and humility. If running like a girl means pursuing this marathon called life with the same awareness as Mina, then in her writing she gives to all of us a fresh pair of running shoes."
—Christopher Harrison, Founder AntiGravity Inc.

"*Run Like a Girl 365 Days a Year* is a fitness roadmap for women. We are all athletes, there is no judgment, and there are no excuses. We just need to move and not look back. Mina Samuels's inspirational thoughts help keep us moving and feeling good about it."

—Nieca Goldberg, MD, Medical Director
Joan Tisch Center for Women's Health

"It often feels like we're stealing—from our jobs, families, and responsibilities—when we take time to run. For the larceny of tending to our bodies and souls, *Run Like a Girl 365 Days of the Year* is an essential accomplice, reminding us daily that the 'stolen' moments may be the ones that matter most."

—Amy Roe, author of *Becoming Boston Strong*

Praise for Mina Samuels

"A chicken soup for the athlete's soul."

—*SELF* Magazine

"There are lots of good sports books, but rarely beautifully written ones. *Run Like a Girl* is both."

—Mary Brophy Marcus, *USA Today*

"A book that is needed and important and life changing—all the things running has been for us!"

—Kathrine Switzer, author of *Marathon Woman: Running the Race to Revolutionize Women's Sports, Running and Walking for Women Over 40*, and co-author of *26.2 Marathon Stories*

RUN LIKE A GIRL 365 DAYS A YEAR

A Practical, Personal, Inspirational Guide for Women Athletes

MINA SAMUELS

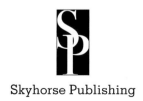

Skyhorse Publishing

CONTENTS

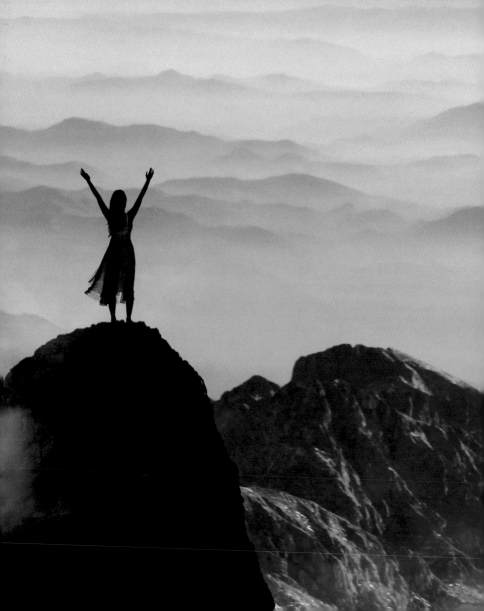

INTRODUCTION

Running like a girl is an everyday experience. Running like a girl happens on the road and off. Running like a girl invites us to engage with the world. Running like a girl means challenging our bodies and minds to be stronger and happier, and accessing our ageless girl-spirit, where the clean-slate optimism of "let's go" meets the seasoned wisdom of "I can."

When I say running, I mean it as a proxy for any active physical engagement you fancy, however you choose to move your body and get your heart pounding! Also when I say running, I mean it as more than a sport. Sports are just one aspect of how we engage with the world as strong women. We have our work, our communities, our families, and our friends; how we are in each of those bits of the world matters.

My first book, *Run Like a Girl: How Strong Women Make Happy Lives*, was about the transformative impact of sports on a woman's life. One of the key currents running through that book was the need for women to renew our commitment to our sports on a continuous basis. A second and equally important undercurrent flowing beneath the pages was that our sports are merely one small piece of our lives.

This book delves more deeply into these topics: How our strength fortifies us; how we find balance; how sports nourish our life's purpose; and how they feed our ability to change how we exist in the world. Our sports are a mirror and microscope. They are where we can test our strength and determination and try out new ways of being.

This book brings together the voices of many strong women I've interviewed and researched, across a range of sports, from running to rugby, from surfing to skating, and dozens in between. But even more, this book is personal. I have been remade by my sports. I have felt the way my strength has supported me on a daily basis and through big changes. At the same time, I struggle with finding the right balance between the supportive potential of my sports and the oversaturation point past which I'm worn out and get injured. I offer this book as a drop of sustenance on this journey we share.

In these pages we will look at serious topics, such as whether this whole business we call life really means anything and how we reach for our dreams, but we will have fun, too. We will revel in the world's beauty. We will laugh at our foibles. Above all, we will contemplate balance, that constantly shifting process of finding our best path in life as strong women.

So this book is a call to be present for the hard work and sweat, and for the joy and indulgence. Know that transforming yourself is a process that doesn't end. Just as water can pass from solid to liquid and then escape the bonds of gravity as a gas, only to return to earth as a raindrop, we too are constantly growing and changing, glimpsing new possibility. And while change may happen quickly, more often it happens over time, even imperceptibly; until one day we realize we are skimming along, legs flying, shoes barely touching the ground.

How to read this book

This book is constructed the way our lives are built—day by day, in a series of daily reflections, often unrelated, always accumulating, which slowly knit together to create each of our unique designs.

You can read this book daily, if you want, but that's not the essential thing. This is *a book of days*, to be read on the days when you are moved to read it. These pages will contemplate how we might approach the world, so that it is a richer, and fuller, happier place; so that it is a place where we can grow and help others grow. "May you go from strength to strength," my father used to wish us on our birthdays and other momentous and liminal occasions. This book is my version of that wish for you.

This is a book to read when you need a boost, when you need a reminder of your worth, or when you question why you run. I don't presume to think that everything I propose in these pages applies to everyone. Take what nourishes you and discard the rest. If something resonates, great. If something annoys you, move on. Or maybe sit with it a second and ask yourself why.

This book is meant to keep you company on this road we are all running. Run strong. Run confident. And run like a girl.

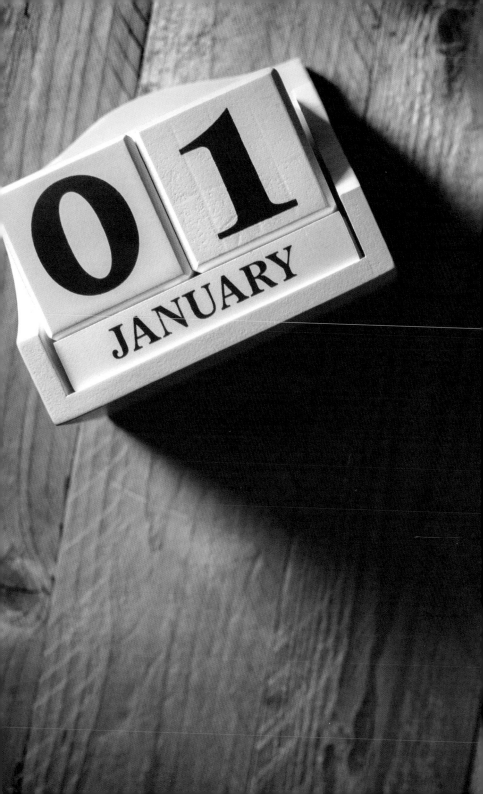

JANUARY

. . . ready, set, GO!

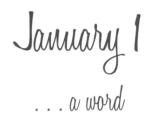

January 1

. . . a word

New beginning. Fresh start.

So much pressure.

Time to distill. What's the one word we would each choose today to describe the year we are aiming for? A word that aspires to something greater, but doesn't set us up for disappointment. A personal word that captures both who we are already and how we can become more. A word that will inspire us for the 364 days to come.

Make a list of possibilities: illuminate, grow, steady, run, light, recharge, strong, vitality, engagement, present, discerning, happy, incandescent, yes, flow, curiosity, change, meet, reliability, spontaneity, pleasure, simplicity . . . These words contain potential.

One year I chose RENEWAL. Another year, I chose ATTENTION.

What's your word?

January 2

. . . grit and grace

For this book, I chose two words: GRIT and GRACE. It's in the space between those words where we run like a girl.

January 3

. . . practice practicing

This year we will be more . . . what?

More intense. More relaxed. More focused. More flexible. More ambitious. More patient.

Whatever it is that we want to be more of, we will have to practice.

And practice practicing.

This year we will practice. More.

January 4

. . . practice opens possibility

I once had a yoga teacher who would say, in moments when she was gently guiding us into a complex origami-shape that required hamstrings five inches longer than mine (i.e., hamstrings that didn't go out running regularly), "It's only practice." A little edgy bit in me sometimes thought, *So when's the actual yoga?*

But actuality and practice are one and the same, of course. The practice is practicing. Getting out on the road for a run is both the run *and* the practice. Most of us can understand intellectually, but we don't always get it at the cellular level. We want our gold star. We want to be done. Completed. Over. Check that box.

Yet we also know that every time we think we've finished something, what we've actually done is practice for the next challenge. A marathon didn't go as well as we'd hoped, so try another one. Or maybe it went better than we could have hoped; where will that trampoline bounce of success take us next?

Practice opens possibility.

January 5

... potentialism

Have you ever tried to stream a movie or TV show and gotten stuck watching the digital circle spinning? Like that circle indicates, there is a good chance (close to 100 percent) that our potential is more than we are currently streaming. Our life takes pauses. The digital circle spins around in the center of our life-screen, trying to catch its tail. That's the sign we need to find a wider bandwidth to stream our full potential.

Not every day is a great run. Not every day will make us feel strong and happy. Even on the not-the-best days of swirl and search, if we can see the *practice* in a slog-of-a-run-through-waist-deep-muck, then we will also see the potential it unleashes.

Let's call that potentialism. But it's not a word, you say? Nope, it's not. It's a neologism, a newly invented word to go with our fresh eyes on a new year.

Potentialism is where we find our widest bandwidth, our deepest connection. More than simple optimism, potentialism is the waking dream, the unconscious made manifest. It's the moment *before* that circle stops spinning on our screen and we see the full picture.

Open to the future. What do you want?

January 6

. . . our life-in-waiting

Potentialism opens our hearts to the future. The actual realization of what we want will not be immediate. We will have a sensation of in-between-ness, of being done with what was, and yet not immersed in what's to come. Our thoughts may feel sluggish and unconnected or rabbit-y and hard to catch.

Our sports give us a structure inside that unsettled state of being. Our bodies give us a way out of our minds. Even as our sports may elevate our spirits, our bodies bring us down to earth, into the raw here-and-now of our flesh, our muscles, our sweat.

If all else feels unripe, unready, in-waiting—our run is ready for us.

January 7

. . . we are 100 percent right now

Amidst all these words of intention, practices, and potentialism, we might get the idea that we are somehow incomplete, an outline waiting to be filled in. Not so.

How many times have you heard someone say, "When I feel like myself again . . ." As in, I'll do such-and-such a thing when I feel like myself again. How can that be? Who are you, if not yourself?

Consider this: What if I will never feel like myself again, because that self I'm waiting to feel like doesn't exist?

I already am myself, and then myself, and myself again. And you are yourself and then yourself, and yourself again.

Every day is different. But we are 100 percent every day. We are enough every day.

January 8

. . . the symphony is playing

As athletes we often feel like our body is a symphony tuning up. That the concert hasn't started yet, that our body is not quite the body it's supposed to be. We are waiting for that magic moment when everything is tuned, and in sync; when all the various aches and pains and injuries and ailments (often a result of our sports) are healed.

I think of myself as a healthy person, but at any given time there is some number of boo-boos I'm monitoring: A skitchy hamstring or a tender hip flexor; an incipient blister on the arch of my foot from an orthotic, plus a hangnail or two; or a persistent crick in my neck.

I've been talking about our bodies, but I could just as easily be talking about anything else in our lives. We are 100 percent and we all have things we are hoping to change or improve. We wonder when the symphony is going to start, when every instrument will play together as it should.

The symphony is already playing. The piece has started and the music is our life as it is right now.

January 9

... why compare?

Your 100 percent is going to look different from someone else's. Guaranteed.

Comparing yourself to others is lose-lose. One road leads to artificial ego inflation and the other to an equally artificial ego deflation. Neither way leads to the truth of you. No one else brings your circumstances to her run. Your best day may be someone else's worst day.

If you must compare, keep your focus on you vs. you.

Practice not comparing. That's easy to write and so very hard for me to achieve. Let's try together.

January 10

... the seventeenth century peacock

A particular passion of mine is translating Jean de La Fontaine's seventeenth century fables from their original French and writing about their contemporary relevance.

Here's a fable about comparing:

The Peacock Complaining to Juno

The Peacock was complaining to Juno,

"Goddess," the peacock said, "it's not without reason that I'm complaining, that I'm muttering. The song you gave me displeases all in nature. Compared to the nightingale, that scrawny weakling, whose sounds are as sweet as they are resonant; to him alone falls the honor of spring herald."

Juno responded in anger,

"Jealous bird, who ought to hold his tongue, is it your place to envy the nightingale's voice? You who wear around your neck a rainbow made of a hundred kinds of silk that glorify you; who deploys a tail so rich that to our eyes it looks like a jeweler's boutique? Is there any other bird under the sun more pleasing than you? No animal has all assets. We have given each of you diverse qualities: Some have grandeur and strength to spare. The falcon is light, the eagle courageous. The raven predicts the future. The crow warns of bad news coming. All are happy with their lot.

So, stop your complaining, or . . . to punish you I'll take away your plumage."

January 11

. . . appreciate what you will miss

Appreciate what you are and what you have. Everything will be taken away sooner or later, if not by Juno, then by time. That's not just a Buddhist-style thought, that's a fact. And you will miss *it*, even if you thought that whatever *it* was wasn't good enough in comparison to others at the time.

Revel in today's run.

January 12

. . . strive for excellence, not perfection

You're not perfect and nobody else is either. Don't waste time comparing. As Carl Jung famously said (and you've probably heard a thousand times, but it bears repeating), "Perfection belongs to the gods; the most we can hope for is excellence."

Excellence is within reach. Excellence is personal. Excellence is an intention, a commitment to manifest your potential. Excellence is putting in our best effort and holding our own selves to our highest standard. Not every action we take is excellent (that's why we practice), but when it's called for, don't hold back the reserves—leave everything on the road (or the field, or in the pool, or . . .) and give it your all. That's it.

What you do won't be perfect. It will be better.

January 13

. . . the voice in our head

There's a little, but persistent, voice in our heads. She's not us, but she is. She can be pretty judgmental, first and foremost of us, but of others, too.

That voice might tell us that our best intentions are stupid, that our potential is limited and possibilities—? More like impossibilities. Our voice might throw out an offhand remark about being fat or ugly or aging. She might try to convince us that we're not up to the task; that we are weak; really, that we're just plain not good enough. Never mind all the *oughts* and *shoulds* she slings around.

She's like the ballerina in our personal music box, and every time we flip the top open (we rarely mean to, yet somehow our finger edges under the lid) there she is spinning around in her tutu, trash-talking us. You're running so slowly today, what's wrong with you?

She's a spin-doctor of the worst kind, mounting smear campaigns and posting attack ads at every opportunity. Even when we think good things about ourselves, she is likely to chastise us for getting cocky, and menace us with the threat that those good qualities will be taken away.

What if we open up her music box, and just let her spin around until she winds herself down? Then we can feel like what we are: strong, warrior rock stars in the hottest girl-band going.

January 14

... not a real athlete

Excerpt of a letter to my parents from McGill University on January 14, 1985: *Rowing has handed out a new training program. I stuck so well to the last one. Anyways they require forty-five minutes of jogging a day plus weights and doing the ergometer machine. Wrong! Actually I went swimming today, not being a real athlete I can't jog in this cold weather and I despise weight rooms.*

The little music box ballerina was spinning dozens of pirouettes the day I wrote that letter.

January 15

... an adult-onset athlete

It took nine more years before the voice in my head stopped telling me I wasn't a real athlete. I've realized now that I am an *adult-onset athlete*. That is, I found a new aspect of myself when I was twenty-eight. Sure, it had always been there. Still, it surprised me.

When we are playing our own original tunes in our warrior girl-band, we have the audacity to try new things. Think new thoughts. Move our bodies in new ways.

So surprise yourself. Try a new sport. No skin in the game. Do it just for the fun of it.

An example: I cross-country ski. Every winter for the past few years I've been telling myself that I'll take a biathlon clinic. Sure, it's an Olympic sport that no one does recreationally, but it looks like just the kind of high-intensity fun I enjoy. Here and now, on this page, I undertake to participate in that biathlon clinic in the winter coming!

January 16

. . . all fun, no work

I once happened upon an exhibit at the Glasgow Gallery of Modern Art called *Blueprint for a Bogey*. In Glasgow, a bogey refers to a homemade go-cart, built from whatever is around, and then driven with reckless abandon by their child-creators. The exhibit was about the idea of play—the way in which we interfere with or restrict children's instinctive desire to play, how we seem to lose our innate ability to play as adults, and how we might reclaim that prerogative.

As adults we are good at burdening ourselves with responsibilities, obligations, and expectations, so that sometimes we feel shackled to our lives. Playing is the opposite. It is free, light, spacious, and unbounded. Play is a creative engagement with the world, without end or purpose.

Yet, as adults, we too often find it challenging to play. Everything we do has to have an agenda; even things that look, at first blush, like play, are, on closer examination, really pursuits in which we are aiming toward a goal—to achieve a certain skill level, to do a race or event, to get fit or lose weight, to win.

We have to pause from time to time and ask ourselves, "Where do I play?"

We need to have play dates with our sports, not just training dates.

January 17

. . . be aimless

I was out playing on my slackline (a tightrope-like piece of webbing, easily secured around two nicely spaced trees) with my partner. A dog-walking woman asked, "Are you training for something?" Her question gave me pause. My only objective was to have fun, to relax, to enjoy hanging out in the park, to lean up against the fat tree and feel the rough ridges of bark digging into my back when it wasn't my turn on the line. Was I being too aimless? Did I need to get more serious?

I am certainly guilty of not playing enough in my sports. I get caught up in wanting to achieve something—to be fitter, faster, more technically skilled. We like to have an answer to the question *why* when we are doing something. We feel uncomfortable if there's no good reason to pursue a particular activity. Add to that that we feel uncomfortable if we aren't good at something. We reach a certain age and think we ought to be accomplished at everything we pursue. We fear looking foolish. How limiting that is.

Playing unfetters us. And what a relief it is to live, even if for only short interludes, in the wide-open expanse of playtime. Play brings more creativity and energy to the rest of our lives.

January 18

... why should my kids have all the fun?

Leslie is an adult-onset athlete and artist. When her kids started playing soccer, she thought, *Why should they have all the fun?* She started playing in an adult soccer league and stuck with it for fifteen years. She'd grown up playing neighborhood sports, swam a bit in college, and practiced some sporadic yoga. Soccer was her first big sports commitment.

She finally had to give it up because she was just getting injured too much. Nowadays she hikes and backpacks and cross-country skis and does yoga and gets to the gym on a regular basis for high-intensity interval training.

The deeper she's gotten into her fifties, the more comfortable she is thinking of herself as an athlete.

January 19

... fit to be a nomad

Leslie has to be an athlete. She's a visual artist whose focus is climate change. She has to be strong and fit to get to the wilderness she photographs—like the Eclipse Icefield, far north in Canada's Kluane National Park.

Her latest project is going back to school. As of 2018, she's enrolled in the University of Hartford's interdisciplinary Nomad 9 MFA; a low-residency program that weaves together curriculum elements around art, ecology, systems thinking, activism, urbanism, and technology. "I wasn't planning on going back to school," Leslie told me. "But it was as if they had designed a program with me in mind, so I had to go back." Surprise.

Leslie isn't just making pretty pictures when she creates art (photographs and encaustic paintings, as well as other media). Her goal is make people more aware with visually and emotionally compelling images. Her athleticism supports her purpose.

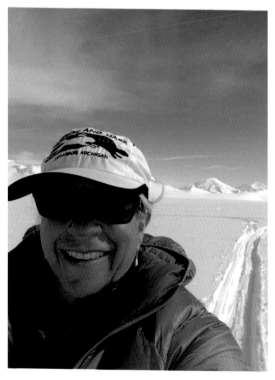

Leslie in Kluane National Park. *Credit: Leslie Sobel*

January 20

. . . our lives have meaning

Some mornings I wake up and wonder if my life has meaning, like after I've talked to someone as passionately engaged as Leslie. Before I've even finished breakfast, I'm wondering why I'm here. Then I'm likely to procrastinate heartily on my to-do list for the day. As if it's better to do nothing at all than to do something meaningless.

But we can all make the world a better place, be good people, and contribute. Our athletics are preparation and practice for that greater work.

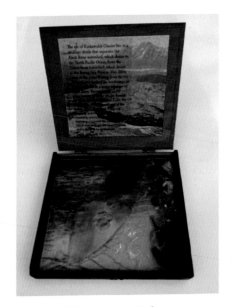

Kaskawulsh Terminus Reliquary.
Credit: Leslie Sobel

January 21

. . . squander your existence

We are here. Our lives have meaning. But let's not get too heavy about it. In *A Preparation for Death*, Greg Baxter wrote, "I spent many years trying to interpret existence, when I ought to have been squandering it."

Practice squandering. Do at least some of your workouts just for fun. Squander kindness and love on people you don't know, or from whom you expect nothing in return. To squander is to live in abundance.

January 22

. . . un-examine

The unexamined life is not worth living.

So said Socrates, by all accounts. And yes, I agree with him, as you can probably guess by now. It would be pretty bold to disagree with a sage of old, wouldn't it?

Except, as in everything, there's a balance to be struck. We may examine our lives so closely that we fall into our own navel. When we over-examine, we are observing when we could be living.

Un-examine sometimes. Stop chasing meaning.

Our sports help us do just this. Even if we are following a strict training regimen, recording all our stats, and keeping logs, our body is going to respond in ways we don't expect sometimes. Because our body—no matter how much we intellectualize, rationalize, explain, or justify—has its own state of being, which, ultimately, we cannot deny. Some days we need to go with the flow we feel inside, literally and physically.

Finding balance is a flow.

January 23

. . . dance

I first heard Zoë Keating's cello piece "Sun Will Set" as I was waiting for a yoga class to start. I was minding my own business, sitting quietly on a foam block with my legs crossed, when I realized that my head and shoulders were dancing. I couldn't stop myself from moving. I hadn't even really noticed the music, until I became aware of its physical effect on me. I tried to hold still, but the pull of the music was too strong. I looked around the room at everyone else—chatting, setting up their props, doing their pre-yoga yoga, napping on their mats—and I couldn't believe they weren't moving to the music. How could they not be drawn into its rhythm? One woman smiled cautiously at me, in the way you smile at people who seem a bit off and from whom you want to keep a distance. Did she even hear the music?

I went home and played the song alone, so that I could dance.

I've started listening to music when I cross-country ski. I discovered that I also love to dance on my skis. Correction: I have no choice but to dance on my skis. Those ear buds cause an involuntary electrical impulse of dance-joy to pass through my nervous system and out through my body. How could my workout not feel better? How could I not feel better?

Dance. More. Whenever. Wherever.

January 24

. . . vegetables and sequins

Liberace once said that too much of a good thing is wonderful. Thomas Paine (the English-American political activist, whose pamphlet *Common Sense* is credited with inspiring the American Revolution) said that common sense is a good thing.

While common sense is a good thing, to be sure, too much common sense is not wonderful. Some days we just don't want to eat our vegetables or get the exercise we need. Of course, Liberace was likely not thinking about common sense, the food pyramid, or target heart rates when he coined that particular phrase. He probably had sex and sequined pantsuits in mind.

So eat your veggies and do your workouts most of the time, but be sure to wear way too many sequins at others.

January 25

. . . expand

Thinking about common sense and sequins reminds us that balance, that Middle Way that Buddhism counsels us to find, is not only about moderation. It is also about expansion. How can we expand into life?

Each year, Edge.org asks a diverse group of cultural, scientific, artistic, and philosophical thinkers to share their so-called last question. One year, Michael I. Norton, a Harvard professor, asked, "Why do humans behave as though what can be known is finite?" Why indeed? Finiteness bounds our awe. Infinity feeds our wonder.

More often than not, the answer to the Big Questions we ask ourselves should be: I don't know. For many of those questions, we can find answers, but even those answers may be mutable, leading to further questions.

In our sports, as it is in life, we must provoke ourselves to expand by asking, asking, asking and trying, trying, trying.

January 26

. . . doing the dishes

Expanding into the Middle Way can sound pretty ethereal.

Here's a Buddhist saying to bring us back from the beyond—
after enlightenment, the dishes.

Also our run.

January 27

. . . micro-progress

Most of us are striving for some earthly version of enlightenment. Searching for the condition in which we have the just-
right, Goldilocks amount of what we need to feel fulfilled, but
we are not so sated that we won't get hungry again.

But really? After enlightenment the dishes (and our run)??
How exhausting. Sometimes just carrying on, one foot in
front of the other, is the challenge we need to rise to on a
given day.

Here's a productivity hack for just getting started: Set
micro-goals. Dopamine-friendly-sized boosts that will keep
you going.

Don't think to yourself: I need to reach a place of perfect
balance, of total equanimity, of complete financial security
and 100 percent good health. Think to yourself, I need to do
these dishes. I need to go for this run. And then I'll see what
might be next on my list.

January 28

. . . moving toward discomfort

Some time ago I took martial arts for a short period (yes, you will notice that in addition to the sports I end up going steady with, there are a lot I've dated casually). The technique that stuck with me was this: if someone attacks you, the best thing to do is to move in the same direction, not pull away. Moving with your attacker will catch him off guard. He will loosen his grip, and, voila, you can snatch your bag back.

Buddhism counsels us to move toward discomfort. To embrace what we are experiencing right now, even if right now is dreadfully uncomfortable and we want nothing more than to be out of the moment. Drawing closer to what we fear may result in more pain in the short term, but ultimately helps us through the moment more than running away ever can.

Life is a marathon for which we can't avoid the training. If we can move alongside the suffering, only then can we loosen its grip.

January 29

. . . the Middle Way

Moving toward the unendurable is nice in concept, but in execution? Sometimes we want to run away and hide from our problems. Sometimes that might seem like a pretty good short-term solution, but like an infection that's never swabbed with alcohol, the problems are more likely to get worse if you ignore them.

Finding our Middle Way is the dance between pulling away from the thief and catching him off-guard by running alongside. Finding balance is the foundation on which we build our lives, so the topic of the Middle Way will recur throughout this book. How do we find balance?, you ask. Lean into a challenge; stand up straight and look it in the eye; lean away. Think through those psychological weight transfers until you find your equilibrium.

The process is like the beginning of a yoga class, when the instructor leads you through a physical version of finding balance. Rock forward on the balls of your feet and back on your heels, then side to side, until you feel the Middle Way in your body. What you do will look different for every sport and will be different every day. We look for the balance in our effort and ease, our focus and openness, our purpose and aimlessness.

January 30

. . . ordinary magic

There is a tree two blocks south of my apartment in New York City that seems to attract an inordinate number of birds. I don't know why the birds love that tree more than others. The avian gathering feels magical.

I once stopped under the tree, gazing up at the birds, angling my phone for a picture. The doorman for the building down the block called out to me, "Don't stand under the birds. You know what birds do!" Indeed. I saw the ground was dotted with bird droppings. I quick-stepped out from under the tree. Magic must meet the ordinary in the end.

Even as we finish a hike through transcendent landscape, we bear fresh bruises, scrapes, and blisters. When we move alongside ordinary discomfort, often we end with magic. The joy of the birds wouldn't be complete without their droppings.

January 31

. . . *bulls and swans*

Speaking of bruises, I bruise easily. Not metaphorically, but literally; as in, purple-black splotches, mostly on my knees and legs, but sometimes on my arms and bum, too. I walk into things with enough frequency that I'm rarely without a bruise. Then there are the bruises from my athletic life. For a period, I rock-climbed quite a bit, and my knees and elbows were constantly covered.

Trail running and *kersplat* have been in a long-term relationship since humans pushed into the upright position and started chasing prey across the veld. In fact, pretty much every activity we do comes with a side portion of bruises. Even if you've never taken ballet (I didn't), we've all seen dancers' feet. We know that, no matter how pretty the performance, strength always has its messy side.

There are days I feel like a bull in the china shop of life. Not only physically, but emotionally and psychologically too. Opening my big mouth. Speaking before thinking. Expressing strong opinions. (Oh what a shrew! How dare she?!)

Our sports prepare us for what is raw in life, for being bulls, even as we are also swans.

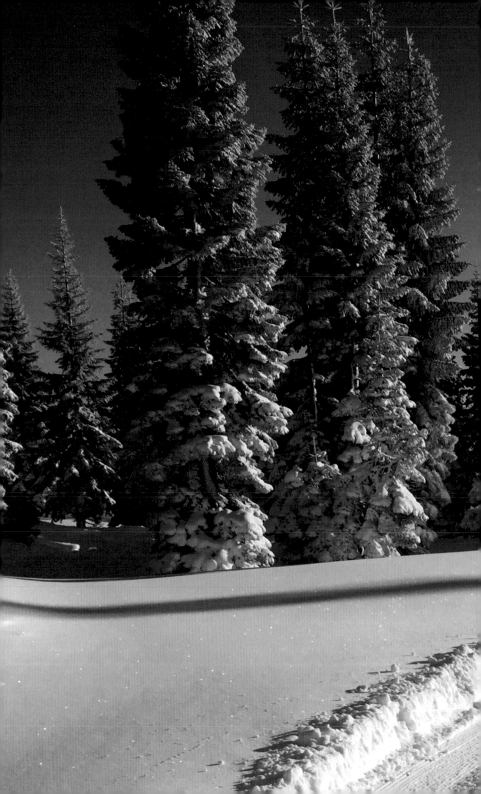

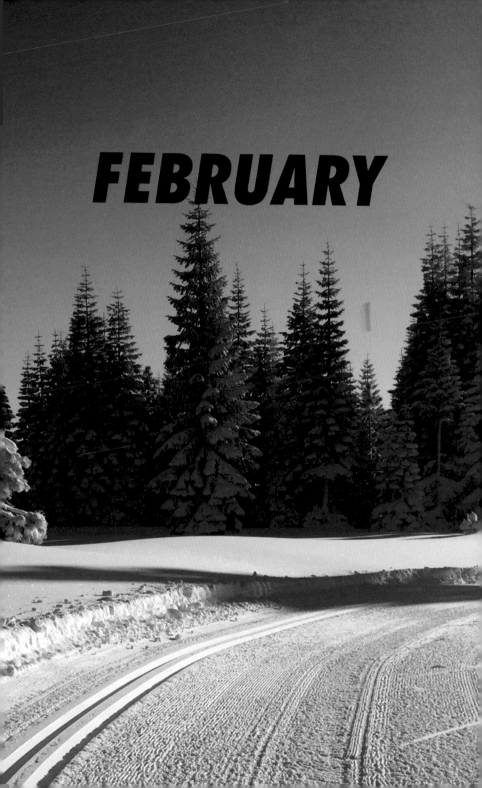

FEBRUARY

February 1

. . . sweat talk

I have a recurring nightmare that I am lost in the maze of halls at the old mansion house of the French school I attended as a young child. In the dream, the headmistress has given me the strap (that's a form of corporal punishment with a leather strap) and I'm desperately trying to get out of the school so my mother can pick me up. In some versions of the dream, I never get out of the school; in others, I get out, only to wait for hours on the front steps, never to be picked up.

A friend of mine's nightmare is a tidal wave that drowns her. More than once she has bitten through the retainer she wears at night.

On the mornings after bad dreams, my surest remedy is to sweat them off. And if I'm lucky enough to have planned my morning workout with a friend, all the better. There's nothing like a good sweat talk (not to be confused with sweet talk, which can be nice on occasion) to peel off the cling-wrap of a bad dream.

To my friends who have shared the roads with me—gratitude and love.

February 2

. . . sleep

I used to think my need for sleep was weak and childish. I'm enjoying that sleep is back in fashion. More and more scientific research suggests that sleep is not just when our brains process, learn, and develop new synaptic connections, but it is also when our muscles repair themselves after the load we've put on them.

When I don't sleep, I feel like one of those ravaged hillsides I've seen in northern British Columbia, those landscapes where the forest has been clear-cut and all that remains is a five o'clock stubble of tree stumps.

When have slept well I feel like a filament of light. *Oh the glory of fresh, clean sheets!*

February 3

. . . my spirit rock

Sleep is not the only time for healing spirits. I have a spirit rock. A giant Sierra boulder, she sits by herself perched above the Euer Valley in Northern California. I don't remember when she first spoke to me.

When I run by her in warm months, I stop and rest my forehead against the warmth of her smooth rock-ness. Press my heartbeat against her chest. From there, I can feel a spiral of energy, pulling my third eye chakra (aka our sixth chakra, the space between the eyebrows) into her, into the earth.

In winter, I rest my palm against her stone skin, brushing off a bit of snow. I always wonder if she will show me something. So far, she hasn't, though I think I can discern patterns in the spiral energy. When I reach for answers with my mind, the spirals dissipate. (How many times will I need to learn that lesson about grasping?)

One time, my partner had gone out skiing earlier. I was skiing with a friend. As we passed my rock, I saw that he had left me a heart, carved into the fresh layer of snow with his ski pole. He knows how much I love my rock.

February 4
. . . rock talk

As much as I love cross-country skiing—the shush speed on snow, the daunting expanse of mountains and sky, the air that feels like biting into a crisp apple—not every day feels as grand as it should. Some days I'm filled with self-hate. My music-box ballerina is foaming at the mouth, because she's talking trash so fast. I can feel her spittle on my face.

One day, early in the season, she was ranting: "You suck. You're no good. You're out of shape. You'll never be in shape again. Why do you even write?" And so on.

I paused at my spirit rock and touched her. I was about to cry. I talked to my rock silently: *I'm sorry I'm such a fuck up.*

I don't know why I can't just enjoy this day. I shouldn't care if I'm not fast enough. Why can't I get over myself?

For the first time, my rock answered me directly. It was not exactly as if she'd spoken *to* me, but as if she had spoken *into* me. She said, "Just leave it all here for now. If you still want all this shit when you pass by again, then you can pick it up."

A lightness bubbled up inside me. I started skiing again, stronger and more easily. Was I faster? *Maybe a little.* Did I feel better? *Much.* A pall that had clung to me for a couple of days dropped away. Just like that. I was so surprised that I kept checking myself. Am I still blue? No. Where did it go? As if I were checking the pockets of my brain to find my lost keys. But I didn't want those keys. The door they opened was gone, at least for the moment.

February 5

. . . rock, shoe, teacup

You could say that my spirit rock was just a voice inside me, that I was speaking to my own self. And you would be right. But not entirely, because I know my rock had something to do with what I heard. How arrogant it would be of me to think that mine is the only voice that speaks inside my head in this vast and mysterious universe. You might say that I endowed the rock with the power to speak to me. If you believe that, we all have the power to endow a rock, a tree, a pair of shoes, a teacup, or a painting with the power to be our positive voice. Even more, we may need that object outside ourselves to hold our better voice for us.

What a power—we can endow an object with the force to show us how to let go. Let's practice that power.

February 6

. . . the Bad Fairy Critic

In a room of fifty women at an event I was speaking at, I conducted a poll. I asked, "How many women here feel good about their bodies?" Only two hands went up, wobbly and tentative. That's 4 percent. Research shows that only 12 percent of women think they look good in a swimsuit. That's three times better, but come on. Both of these numbers are ridiculously low. Is this really how we want to live—in a state of perpetual discomfort about our bodies? Of course not.

There's a critical insight in that 8 percent disconnect between the hesitant hand-raisers together in a room with me and the beach-bound, bikini set in an anonymous research cohort. It's likely that those 12 percent who felt good in their swimsuits didn't openly proclaim that sentiment with pride. Oh no, they were answering questions on an anonymous poll for a study on women and body image. It's easy to be honest when you're not identified.

I wouldn't raise my hand in a room full of women, even if I felt good about my body that day. Why? Because I'd be fearful that all the other women in the room would be raising their mental eyebrows and telepathically communicating with each other, *That girl feels good about herself? With that flat chest?*

You know what I'm talking about, don't you? You've met that Bad Fairy Critic (BFC) inside you who spends all her time sizing up other women. We all have.

Can we just stop?!

February 7

. . . BFC-proof earplugs

When it comes to body talk and our BFC (remember her from yesterday?), we women aren't doing each other, or ourselves, any favors. We are in a vicious cycle, which we perpetuate every time we see a friend and say, "You look great, have you lost weight?" Or, "You're so slim." Or we say, "I just need to lose however-many pounds." Take time to notice for a few days how utterly common it is in the course of a conversation for women to comment on their own, and each other's, bodies. We think this is an acceptable, interesting, or worthy topic for us to expend our energy on.

Guess what? For the most part, the topic is not worth the breath. When someone tells us we look slim, we feel good . . . for a nanosecond. Until it settles in that someone is noticing how we look, and then we start to worry about whether we'll measure up the next time. Because we know that we're doing the very same thing right back at other women. In the end, that BFC is just like our music-box ballerina, only she projects our own insecurities onto others. Round and round and round we go.

The good news is we can put in our special BFC-proof earplugs. Breathe some fresh air, unpolluted by the noxious gas of body talk. Let's compliment our sisters on their vitality, achievements, energy, and compassion.

February 8
... start with noticing the BFC

Like much else, quieting the BFC starts with noticing. Over the years I have, at various times, committed to no more body talk. It's hard. One time I lasted only four paltry hours. Deciding whether my friend's arms looked better in a particular dress than mine did derailed my intention. I've re-resolved. And re-resolved again.

I've realized the task is to notice, just notice, how often body talk comes up in conversations with friends, acquaintances, and colleagues, and in our own heads. When do you notice her most? Is she quieter or louder when you're doing sports? Practice plugging your ears with intent.

February 9
... an idea of an office

Somewhere along the early road of my life, another, completely different voice in my head told me that a proper office must be accessed by an elevator, in a tall building, where the windows didn't open, and secretaries glided around hushed halls. When I was growing up my father didn't go to a *real* office for work. His law-professor office was more like a library with a desk, located in the semi-basement of an old stone building. My two younger brothers and I would visit my dad by climbing into the window well, tapping on the leaded glass panes to make our presence known, and waiting for my dad to crank open the window.

I don't know where I got my idea about offices and what they ought to be like. My mother was a weaver and co-owned an artisan craft shop. One of my grandfathers was an apple farmer and the other was in the family department-store business in Regina, Saskatchewan. But this idea of the elevator and tall building so infected my conception of what constituted success that I pursued the ideal as my own, until I realized it wasn't anything I actually wanted.

That's where running made its entrance.

February 10

. . . windows should open

Now, even with their great air circulation and sweeping, spacious views, I feel as if I'm suffocating in big corporate offices, with all that glass and granite and windows that don't open.

For a time in my life I practiced law at a high-powered firm, and every day I swooshed up an elevator in a coldly marbled building. Even the receptionist seemed to be made of marble. It was not a happy time. I had an interior office. This was before the architectural design concept of shared light. I often lived in an artificial-light environment for days on end, arriving at work before the sun rose and leaving after sunset. In boardroom meetings or partners' offices I would gaze longingly out the windows, trying to absorb as much natural light, before burrowing into the interior again. But even with glimpses of natural light, I craved real air too, even if it was cold or hot or damp or polluted.

My workouts were snatched at the gym in the same building. I don't remember windows, only televisions. Then running hit my bloodstream.

I left the practice of law. Besides the mal-illumination, there were other mismatches with my temperament.

Important lesson learned: Windows should open.

February 11
. . . the first two loops

I moved from Toronto to New York City in 1993 to pursue a masters of law degree at Columbia University. I was on a leave of absence from that law firm of closed windows. I started running a few days a week, making my way out and back along parts of the perimeter of Central Park. I was too scared to go into the actual park. When I finally got up the courage to venture inside the park, I was struck. Well hello, there were so many other runners. Buoyed by their energy, I built up my mileage. A few months in, I was running a whole loop of the park in one go—about a 10K.

I was quite pleased with myself. When a woman I knew

to be a marathon runner asked me how much I ran, I said, "Oh, I run about ten, three times a week." The woman was more impressed than I expected. I walked away with an extra shot of pride zinging through my veins, until I remembered. I was in the United States, not Canada. The US thinks in miles, not kilometers.

I had never run ten miles in one go. Ever. I went back to my apartment. Put on my running gear. Went out to Central Park. Ran two loops. Wondered where the woman inside of me who could do that had come from.

Felt windows opening all around me.

February 12
. . . don't take ordinary for granted

So many years have come and gone since that day. The idea of running two loops of Central Park feels ordinary now. Not an everyday thing, to be sure, but still, not unusual, not life changing. I'm a runner now. It's practically like sleeping and eating and breathing. Sure, there are periods when running hasn't been available to me. I've been sidelined by injuries. Or I'm in a place where running isn't possible. Over the years, I have cut back on the number of running days in favor of more cross training. But no matter, I'm always a runner.

Sometimes I almost forget that running changed my life. That running blew the top off my head, shattered window-glass in my mind, and opened my heart to new possibility. That it launched me in a new direction, from practicing law to writing.

I almost forget, but not quite. Then, running on a rainy day in winter, I'll remember—this is hard; this is special; this is transformative—the heat of my sweat hits the chill air, liquid becomes gas, steam rises off my clothes as my energy is released into the world.

February 13

. . . get started already

"For a long time, it had seemed to me that life was about to begin—real life. But there was always some obstacle in the way, something to be got through first, some unfinished business, time still to be served, a debt to be paid. Then life would begin. At last it dawned on me that these obstacles were my life."

This quote is credited to Alfred D'Souza, who was perhaps an Australian philosopher, maybe even theologian, who died in 2004. Nobody in Google-land knows for sure. How refreshing! Whoever this person was, he (she? they?) offered thoughts out to the world with no need for credit, no product tie-in, and no desire for accolades.

The quote rings familiar. Like ancient wisdom repackaged. We might think we don't need to hear it again. Yet, if we're honest with ourselves, there was probably sometime in the last hour (maybe even five minutes), when we thought to ourselves, *when X happens, then I'll be happier, more fulfilled*, by which we somehow mean, more alive.

Not happening. We will never be more alive than we are right now. Let's stop setting conditions on our aliveness. Let's stop belittling ordinary everydayness. What if we just let our energy rise up into the world?

February 14

. . . a valentine for my body

I woke up this morning intending to go for a run. Yesterday was my day off. The sun was shining for the first time in what felt like weeks. I was alone, listening to the silence in my apartment with my cat nestled on the pillow beside me. I was thinking about a friend who had thrown out her back trying to move a heavy piece of furniture in her mother's empty apartment and how obvious it seemed to me that her back was telling her to stop torturing herself over the family politics involved with the apartment.

I started to think about getting up and out on the road for a run. That was when my body began to talk to me. First it pointed out to me that I seemed quite eager to interpret what my friend's back pain was saying to her, while pretending not to hear my own body. My body continued speaking, not scolding, just drawing my attention to a few things. Like how tired my legs felt just lying in bed. How sore my feet were. How the little ache in my back piped up every time I rolled over. My mind started to answer back with its usual blandishments, but my body cut it off. Not today, my body explained. Today, we are going to try something new—a second day off in a row.

This extra day of rest is a valentine to my body. Sometimes getting started means resting.

February 15

... two days off

The last time I took two days off in a row was over a year before that Valentine's Day. I'd had surgery for a neuroma in my foot. The surgery was early on a Friday morning, so I couldn't workout beforehand. I did nothing on Saturday either. On Sunday, I rode a Citibike (a shared social bike system in New York City) with a surgical boot on my foot. Not a workout, but not immobility either.

Disciplined. Obsessive. Each of those labels may apply, depending on the day. The point is—I will talk about rest in this book. A lot. But I must tell you that I am not very good at resting. Sleeping, yes. Resting, not so much. I want to be better.

February 16

... right effort

In his book, *Advice Not Given: A Guide to Getting Over Yourself,* Mark Epstein, a psychiatrist and practitioner of Buddhism, describes right effort, a concept that seeks the middle ground between asceticism and materialism. Both are manifestations of our ongoing wrestling match with our egos. When we exert too much energy (whether it is in self-denial or in consumption) we will be restless, anxious, and unfocused.

When we spend too little energy, we will be lax, careless, and foggy. When we learn to relate to our egos in a balanced way, we relate to our egos in a new way. "It is here that we can apply the analogy to athletes finding *the flow* when they learn to get out of their own way," Epstein writes.

Taking a second day off in a row was the right effort for my body that day. It might not be another time. I have to experiment. Exploring the changing boundaries of right effort is an essential step in the dance of finding our balance.

Trying new things is not always about exertion. Often, it must be about taking the foot off the gas.

February 17

. . . first date anniversary

Today is the anniversary of my first date with my partner. On a mild winter evening in 1994, we met for a run. Our loop around Central Park turned into dinner together in our running clothes, plus a sweatshirt of his that I borrowed before dinner to ward off the post-sweat chills.

Fast forward through thousands of runs and dinners. Our running fashion changes with the times, shorts of different lengths, some skirts (for me), minimalist and maximalist shoes. Roads give way to trails. We add cross-country skiing and mountain biking. The restaurant where we ate our first dinner closes and reopens as something new multiple times. Different signs hang out front. My hair is long and short and various shades of red. We each cycle through injuries, recoveries, and returns to running.

The years inscribe themselves. We still meet for runs, at our shared front door.

February 18

. . . not enough time

I saw an interview with Tilda Swinton where the actress discussed playing an immortal vampire in Jim Jarmusch's film, *Only Lovers Left Alive*. She talked about imagining the mindset of immortality as never having to sweat the small or big stuff, because you had all the time in the world.

I don't feel like I have all the time in the world. Maybe in some karmic "we-live-more-than-one-life" scenario I do. But this Mina-human who is sitting at her desk writing now, feels like she has this one shot. She gets anxious about missing a workout. What if that sunny day when I took a second day off in a row was the last day of sunshine?

You may not have exactly the same thought. But I would go all-in on a bet that you have some version. That's our egos, convinced that if we exert enough energy we will bring death to its knees. Then, like vampire-Tilda, we won't have to sweat the small or big stuff.

We are athletes, not vampires. We like to sweat. And our bodies need rest.

February 19

. . . insatiability

Rachel didn't start figure skating lessons until she was twelve years old. She trained with another girl who went on to become a gold medalist, but that girl started her training younger. As

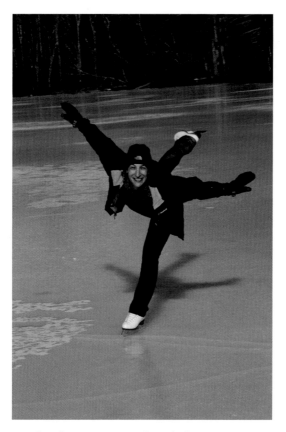

Credit: Photo courtesy of Rachel

much as Rachel secretly dreamed of an Olympic medal, she also knew she started training too late. The experience left Rachel with a lifelong insatiability, a feeling like there isn't enough time for all the things she wants to accomplish, on and off the road. She's accomplished a lot—triathlons, marathons, backcountry skiing adventures, vice presidency of new distribution channels at a major media company.

Her running has been sidelined by multiple injuries, but her insatiability drives her to set other goals—multi-peak hikes in the Adirondacks, doing a freestanding handstand, starting her own business one day, creating an engaged and compassionate environment for her children to flourish. She's always figuring out new ways to raise her game.

Rachel has been getting up in the morning for a sport since she was twelve. Now in her early forties, she won't be stopping anytime soon.

February 20

. . . pretend you've smoked a joint

Once when Rachel was heading onto the rink to try landing the double lutz, her figure skating coach said, "Rachel, pretend you've smoked a joint. Now go try the double lutz."

Rachel didn't smoke pot, but she knew what her coach meant. Relax. Give it everything you've got. Being high makes it easier to see the deep harmony in those last two sentences, instead of the surface clash. Rachel landed that double jump.

Whether she's about to go into a challenging meeting, or

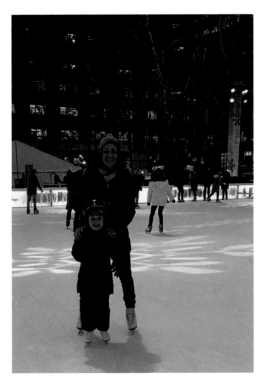

Credit: Photo courtesy of Rachel

about to ski down an untracked pitch, Rachel thinks about her coach's advice.

February 21

. . . the danger of self-fulfilling prophesies

Rachel recently started doing a new high-intensity interval workout in the CrossFit style, involving a mix of cardio, weight lifting, gymnastics, and core training. She's noticed that a lot of the people in the class get all worked up before the class even starts, talking smack, psyching themselves out with self-directed messages that the class will be too hard and they won't be able to do it.

I do that too sometimes. I've noticed that when I convince myself in advance that I'm not up to something, I usually end up fulfilling that prophecy. At aerial Pilates, on the days I think, "Today I can't do all the core exercises," invariably I don't. But if I say to myself, "Today is the day I'm going to do all of them." I get a lot closer to 100 percent. Maybe one day I'll be strong enough to do every crunch to the max, not to mention all the other challenges I'd like to master.

Our minds are the key to any challenges we face, both in our sports and in the world. If we can relax in the midst of our focus, we can elevate our performance.

February 22
... the Philosopher-Trainer

We live in an age of the Philosopher-Trainer. On any given day, in any flavor group workout, in addition to the usual "fight for it," "just ten more," and "you can do it," we are also likely to hear that we are transforming ourselves with each pedal stroke, with each asana, with each Pilates-hundred. Our Philosopher-Trainer tells us that the mere fact of our getting stronger will make us happier, and therefore make the world a better place.

Sounds simple. Sounds improbable. It is not enough to serve ourselves big doses of pleasure to make the world better. Yes, there's the oxygen mask that we all need to put on first, before we can be helpful to anyone else. After all, we need to be breathing to make a contribution. And our contribution must go beyond the Philosopher-Trainer's quasi-spiritual encouragement.

How can I bring my energy into the world as a positive force today?

February 23

. . . wu wei

The Taoist principle of *wu wei* captures our task in a paradox described as the "action of non-action." *Wu wei* asks us to cultivate a state of being in which our actions align with rhythms and cycles of the natural world. When we do, then our actions (or non-actions) will be effortless, offered in service of the greater good, in flow with the universe.

We can learn to feel the flow of the universe in our sports. Then we are better able to bring that non-action out into the world with us. If all that sounds a bit mumbo-jumbo—think of Rachel's coach and imagine that you've just smoked some pot. When we act from that place of ease, we offer our right effort to our fellow travelers.

February 24

. . . another word for purpose

The flow of *wu wei* begins from the core of our natures as human beings inextricably connected to each other, to animals and other living things, to the energy of the universe.

But we humans like to have more concrete terms to hang on to other than *flow* and *connection* and *core*. Why am I here? Why are you here? What is the word that describes your purpose and the core of your nature?

Mine is BELONGING. The word was given to me (by the universe, by my guides) during a vision quest I did some years ago in the New Mexico desert (more on that next month). My purpose word guides me in my work. This book was born during the time I spent in the desert. I wrote it because I wanted to share my reflections on how each one of us belongs and how our sports can ground us in that belonging.

So now we have two words. What is the conversation between your word of the year and your purpose word?

February 25

. . . turpitude

Turpitude is such a great word that I want to include it in this book for its zest. It came to mind because I was thinking about purpose and what its opposite might be. When we act or don't act with purpose, we are attending to something greater than ourselves, therefore its opposite is more than purposelessness; it is to act not only against others' interests, but against our own.

That's the essence of turpitude, a word whose root derivation is shame. Why would we want to do something shameful? Shame does not flow. It jams us up. Locks us down. We lose our way inside of shame.

When I do or don't do something that causes another person (or even me) to feel like they don't belong, I lose my sense of direction. Purpose provides a map back to our selves. Our sports give energy to our purpose.

February 26

. . . re-finding our purpose

We will lose our way.

Every time I think I have found my meaning, the *why* of why I'm here, it slips from my grasp. I've told you that belonging is my purpose word. But hanging onto certainty of purpose is like holding wind—if we reach for it, it will escape; if we hold our hand out, it will caress our outstretched palm. Even as I write this book, my fingers will tighten around an idea I want to convey. For the umpteenth time I have to unclench my hand.

Trust that you are still here with me. Trust that we are finding our way together.

February 27

. . . zeal and forgiveness

It's hard to be a good person in the world, to always know what the right thing is to do. Because the thing is, I want to have fun too, to not be so zealous that I alienate others.

We all need to forgive ourselves more, to internalize the idea that it's okay if we don't get everything right. How else could I ever be willing to let these pages out into the world?

February 28

. . . we are not separate from one another

I feel the truth of the Buddhist idea that we are all connected. That we are not the separate individuals we think we are; that our *self* is a delusion, which cuts us off from others; that what we do matters to other people; that it reverberates throughout the world.

Our workouts nourish our best selves, yes. Then we can plant our energy in the world with how we act. From how we treat our nearest, to how we treat the stranger we instinctively dislike, to our work, to our care for the planet and all its living creatures—one act at a time.

February 29

. . . interconnectedness

"I . . . a universe of atoms . . . an atom in the universe."
—Richard Feynman

The theoretical physicist reminds us that we are connected to everything and everything to us.

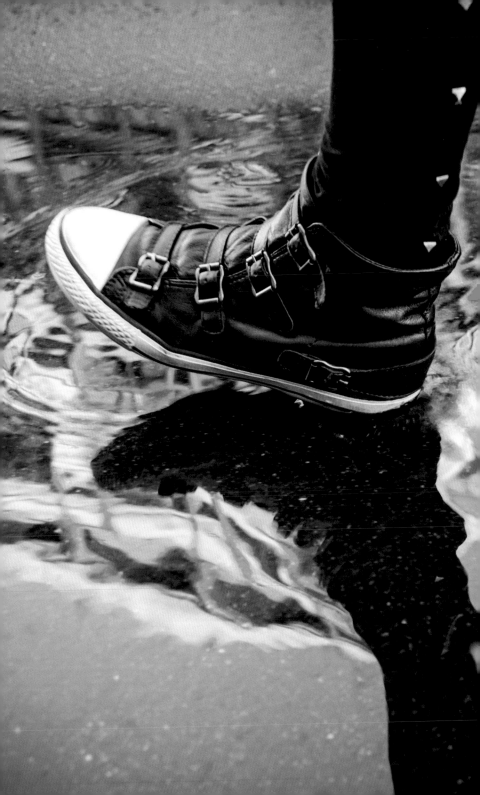

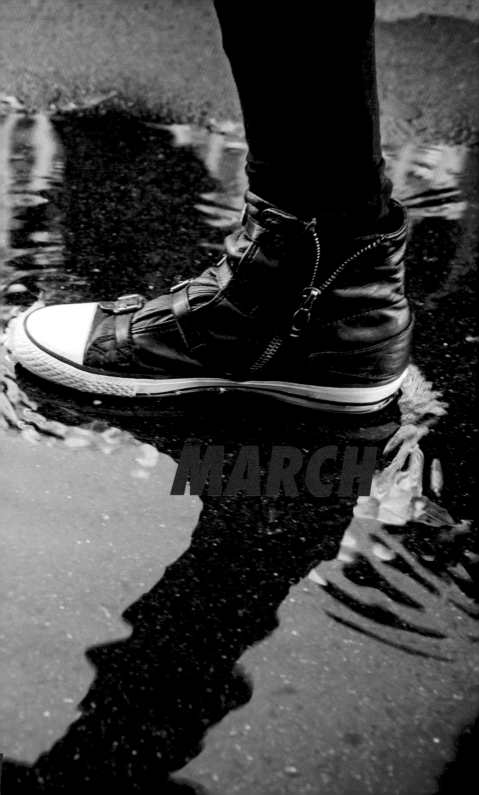

MARCH

March 1

... like a lamb

As much as I love cross-country skiing, the beginning of March is about the time I start to think about hanging up my skis for the year. Even if March is going in like a lion, dumping snow on any over-eager daffodils, I can hear the roads and trails starting to clear their throats.

I love the seasons for the way they impose themselves on us, demanding that we adjust to their temperament in how we dress and what we do, keeping us nimble, keeping us alert.

March 2

... the wind in your face

One of my favorite runs takes me up the west side of Manhattan to the George Washington Bridge and the little red lighthouse nestled below. The route is an out and back, and yet, too often, the wind is in my face in both directions! It doesn't seem meteorologically possible, never mind the metaphoric implications that come with a headwind in all directions.

The wind will not always be at our backs. We can choose to fight tooth and nail against the wind, which just is; or we can enjoy the breeze.

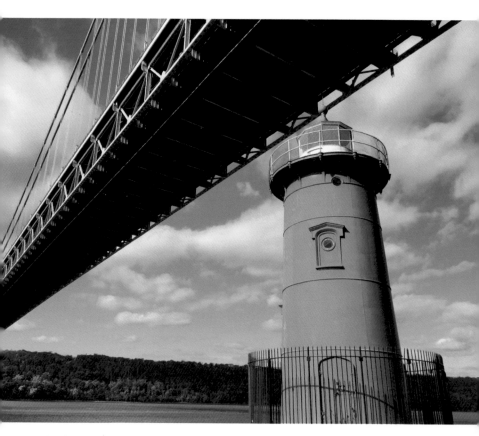

The little red lighthouse beneath the George Washington Bridge in Upper Manhattan. *Credit: Mina Samuels*

March 3

. . . physical pain

I realized recently while trying to describe a particular pain to a doctor, that I could distinguish between quite a few different kinds of physical pain: the hot-sharp, then diffusing, pain of a broken bone; the cattle-prod jolt and tingle of nerve pain; the bruise-ache of an irritated fascia; the sting of a deep cut; the sparkle of inflamed-nerve electricity; the tingle-jangle that zips up a leg as an acupuncture needle penetrates. So much pain, all different. And I haven't even gotten to psychic and emotional pain.

Yet without pain, how would we know what comfort felt like?

March 4

. . . the injury cornucopia

The list of running injuries I've dated, or had long-term relationships with, keeps getting longer. Plantar fasciitis, which manifests as pain in my heel, but actually emanates from issues in the arch of my foot, has hung out with me on and off for more than a decade. A Morton's neuroma, a sensational nerve pain between the third and fourth toes, lived with me for about six increasingly electrical years until I finally had the blasted nerve surgically removed (*hallelujah*). My left hamstring enjoys making me squirm when I sit for long periods. I've had casual relations with pain in my IT band, my shins, my hip flexors, and a few other passing acquaintances I've forgotten.

I've been shot up with cortisone (unhelpful) and PRP (worked the first time, not the second—it was experimental on neuroma, still worth a try); had acupuncture, electrical shockwave therapy, and laser therapy (efficacious, but not quite enough). I've worn orthotics (hello blisters and no relief); engaged in different stretching and strengthening protocols (sticking with it is always the challenge); gotten intimate with various rollers (hurt me so good and for those who are lucky enough not to know what that is—it's a cylinder one sits or lies on top of to use body weight to roll over knotted muscles); and I'm surely forgetting a few other things.

Staying on the road is never guaranteed. I know I need to be grateful for every day I am. Easier said than done. I set that intention and reset, and again.

March 5

. . . tantric running

On this morning's run I was trying to practice the Tantra, as I understand the concepts from dharma talks. The practice (as applied to running—I'll leave you to read up on tantric sex yourself) is to notice what I am enjoying and simply attend to the joy, luxuriate in it, feel it fully, and, of course, not get attached to it. The weather was Goldilocks-perfect.

Not too hot. Not too cold. The sun was shining. The air was that fresh-and-clean that follows a torrential rainstorm. The New York skyline was sharp and clear as the first day in new eyeglasses, when the whole world comes into focus again. I started out tired and dragging, but somewhere along the way I picked up some energy. I was starting to glide.

But, this whole non-attachment business is difficult. In the midst of the bounty, I was struck by a wave of melancholy at the thought that a day will more than likely come when I may never run again. I wanted to be sure to store the joy away, so that when that day did come, I could still open a cupboard in my memory and get a whiff of it again.

I attached. It's hard to feel joy without wanting to hang on to it. I need to keep working on this whole non-attachment business. Gently uncurling my grasping fingers.

March 6

. . . clean public bathrooms

I began a personal campaign a few years ago to leave public bathrooms in a better state than when I arrive. This most often involves picking up bits of paper towel and toilet paper from the floor. I do it as a form of personal-karma cleanup. Bathrooms along running routes are among the worst.

When I was interviewing for my first law job, long before my public bathroom project, I was wined and dined by a few firms. At one swish restaurant, as the maître d' pulled out my chair, I noticed that a napkin from the previous diners had fallen on the floor. I picked it up. One of the lawyers said, "You should have let the maître d' pick that up."

I made the mistake of signing on with that law firm. But then again, that experience helped me out of the practice of law and onto the roads and then onto this page.

March 7

. . . running like a girl into theatre

My post-law life as a runner and writer has undergone its own transformations. While I was working on my first *Run Like a Girl* book, I became friends with a man who introduced me to several of the women I interviewed. It was he who provoked me onto a stage.

Theatre was my passion into my teens. I had put it away for a long time, but when I mentioned my long-lost love to this new friend, he said, "Well why don't you sign up for a theatre class?" When I tried to explain that New York was too competitive for me to take a theatre class, he just raised his eyebrows. He might as well have said, "I dare you." I have, as you already know, a bit of a tendency to jump in.

The woman who taught the first class I signed up for is now a close friend. She was my director for the two solo shows I wrote and performed and a collaborator on an ensemble show I wrote. I did a workshop around that play at Western, the university in my hometown in Canada, and befriended two amazing theatre professors. They were visiting New York on the day I signed this book's contract. That felt like the world completing a rotation.

Each transformation builds on the previous one, cycling back around to gather the threads together again. Every day contains all the past days. Time loops. It's 1993. I am in Central Park again, running twice round for the first time.

March 8

. . . inundated by aphorisms

Relentless aphorisms litter every legible, exposed surface of one of the ubiquitous re-usable shopping bags I see everywhere these days; bags which have become a fashion accessory in and of themselves.

Dance, sing, floss, and travel. To move forward in life, forgive your parents for everything you think they did wrong. Drink water. Do yoga. Sweat. Do one thing a day that scares you.

Does it have to be every day? I like to be outside my comfort zone. But on some days I like it only a little (or not at all).

We don't need to be full-on scared every day. Some days we can give our hearts a break.

March 9

. . . not too glib

From my ultra-fallible, personal mountaintop it seems like a wave of easy-as-1-2-3 spirituality is washing through the world's thinking. Everywhere I turn people are tossing off Zen-esque speak, the way my grandmother would throw a pinch of salt over her shoulder as a meal was starting, for health and luck.

Let's not get too glib with our talk of spirit and transformation. If the homilies move inside our comfort zone, then we will lose track of the real, hard, continuous effort that is required to be present to the hardcore demands of change and transformation. Life is a marathon (if we're lucky!). Have I said that before? Yes. Will I say it again? Yes. There's no "one and done" in our pursuit of living our fullest life.

March 10

. . . strict diets

For some years I maintained vegan Sundays. I discovered that strict diets (veganism felt quite restrictive) are hard to maintain, unless you lead a monkish existence, or have friends who have identical eating habits. Eventually I stopped my vegan Sundays. It turns out I eat vegan considerably more than three meals a week already—there was no need to hold myself to a strict schedule. Being easy with others was more important to me.

Just as our workouts can go stale, our priorities can call for a reset. Our task is to test, keep, or discard, repeat from the beginning. Despite what I said yesterday about glibness and hardcore-ness, not everything has to be hard.

March 11

. . . generative adversarial networks

Generative adversarial networks (GANs) are one of the new frontiers in deep learning. When I first encountered the expression "deep learning," I felt like it summed up an excellent life philosophy and a new angle on this knotty issue of finding balance. Plus, who doesn't want to learn profoundly?

GANs are deep neural-net architectures comprised of two opposing sides. I read about them in the context of a technology that generated fake faces. Disturbing, I know, but let's set that aside for now. One of the neural nets (the generator) generates fake faces (digital images that appeared to be real people), sending thousands of its iterative efforts to its adversary (the second neural net). That second neural net (the discriminator) detects fakeness. For every fake detected, the first neural net tried again. Each system learned how to do its job better. The faker generated better fakes. The fake-detector became more discriminating.

This same scenario can apply to each of us in life. Every day, life is giving us feedback on how we are doing. We can receive the wisdom and learn from it, or (not to be glib) we can keep on doing the same thing over and over, expecting different results.

March 12

. . . listen to life

Listening to what life is telling us can be hard. What is it really saying? Sometimes it seems like life is trying to discourage us. Life rarely feels over-encouraging, but if and when it does, lucky you. Does a discouraging response mean you should try something different, or just try harder? It means try both, if possible. Learn. Rinse and repeat.

Our workouts are their own GANs. Are you someone who always follows a rigorously scheduled itinerary of workouts? What if you didn't for a week? What if you just did what your body asked for? Are you someone who hates to plan workouts in advance, because you want to wait and see how you feel? What if you set up a specific schedule in advance and stuck to it no matter what for a week? Is a week long enough for either of these experiments?

Generate. Discriminate. We can always be learning.

March 13

. . . reassess and then again

I believe in the transformative impact of sports on women's lives. Most days. Because I have to admit that there are some days when I think that instead of making us strong and happy, running or exercise operates as a distraction, a substitute addiction, a new way to avoid looking inside ourselves, and a new thing to beat ourselves up about.

We can use our sports to get to know ourselves or to hide from ourselves. We have to investigate what's true for us, and that's a process that requires continuous calibration and honesty. Assess. Reassess. Again.

March 14

. . . my one sports team

I was only ever on one sports team in my life—volleyball in high school. I sat on the bench. Every game. Except one. It was the game that happened the night after a big party, to which I wasn't invited. There was a direct relationship between popularity and first-string of the volleyball team. Being unpopular, I was one of the only players not hung over, and so got a chance to play my only game.

Since then, I've built my own team: my workout partners; writers with whom I share my work; theatre collaborators; and my friends and family. These are the people who won't leave me on the bench. I am grateful for my team and love them with my whole heart.

March 15

... beware the ides

Poor Julius Caesar, his team could have just left him on the bench. Instead they betrayed him. Changing the course of Roman history.

March 16

... thoughts just are

The vision quest I once participated in was a twelve-day program of all women, led by two guides. We spent four days sitting in what's called a council circle, sharing and refining the intention we brought with us to reflect on. This was followed by a four-day fast and period of contemplation alone in the New Mexico desert. Then we returned for four final days to tell our stories and absorb the teachings of each of our journeys.

One evening, as I was meditating in solitude out in the desert, watching the sky for the appearance of the first star, I found my mind wandering: *If I type in black lace bandeau on Amazon.com, will the search results come up with what I want to solve the way a new favorite blouse gaps open at the front? Will it ship in two days free with my Prime account? Or will it be one of those Amazon partners, who ship in their own sweet time?*

I caught myself, and berated myself for being shallow. I had a lot of time and space to berate. More time passed and I saw the bandeau was just a thought. My only task was to have a look at what my mind was up to, not judge its contents.

Anyway, who decides what the right thoughts at the right time are anyway? The main thing is to practice finding the pause to notice.

March 17

. . . empathy

It was on that same vision quest in New Mexico that I learned how to make that uniquely female sound—the low, guttural hum of agreement and sympathy, which comes from deep in the back of our throats. Until then, I had envied the resonance of those women who could express their empathy with a sound that carried such soothing weight, but I could never bring myself to make it. It felt false in my throat.

Mmmmhmmm.

Listening to the hard stories many of the women at the quest had to share, there in the parched, hot sun, I found myself, without conscious intent, making the sound. The universal sound of "I hear you, sister. I understand. And I feel it too." You can make the sound for your workout partner, when you are sharing woes. You can even make it for yourself. I admit it. I verbalize to myself on long solo workouts.

Empathy hurts, even as it heals. We need the sound to release the shared pain.

March 18

. . . racquet sports

Trigger warning: I had a tennis instructor once . . . well I only ever had one tennis instructor . . . who forced me to give him a blowjob when I was fifteen. I had a crush on him, yes, but I was a girl at the time and he was a man. When he offered to take me for ice cream, I wanted the ice cream, not to be taken to his house, where I was too scared to say no to anything he asked.

I never did learn how to play tennis. After that, I quit the lessons and never told my parents why. I pretended to have lost interest, which they believed, since at the time they viewed me as a pretty disengaged teen.

I tried learning squash in university, but that instructor was like an octopus, his hands everywhere, when showing me how to hold the racquet. I thought it must be my fault that I couldn't take racquet lessons without inciting some kind of impropriety.

I wish I didn't have so much company in this experience. Belatedly, #MeToo helped me see who was behaving poorly. Hint, it wasn't me. It's taken me years to realize that.

March 19

. . . a champion's resilience

At a conference in 2012 on women and sports, Diana Nyad spoke. She is a world-renowned long-distance swimmer. At sixty-three, after five attempts (since the 1970s), she became the first person to swim the 102 miles from Florida to Cuba without a shark-protection cage. Just from that, you can get an idea of her zeal and commitment to the sport.

At this conference she spoke for the first time (this was well before #MeToo) about the sexual abuse she had suffered at the hands of her grade-school swim coach.

At the time, I wondered: *If I were a more resilient person, would I have become a champion at racquet sports?* Well that was a potential black hole of a thought; using another woman's resilience to beat up on myself. Then I remembered—I didn't even like tennis that much to begin with.

March 20

. . . runny nose

For me, resilience often involves a runny nose. When I get nervous, in particular when I'm on stage, my nose starts to run. My runny nose never happens in rehearsal alone with the director, but as soon as other people come to watch, I'll feel the thin dribble run down my upper lip. What to do? I'm on stage.

My nose also runs when I'm running or cycling. Something about the effort and the outdoor air, I think. Or is it nerves? It's possible. For some reason, no matter how many thousands of times I've gone running or cycling, I almost always feel a subtle undercurrent of *can-I-do-this?*

Is my runny nose a sign that I'm just outside my comfort zone? If so, that's probably right where I want to be. Our comfort zone is for resetting, before we venture out. Again.

March 21

. . . consistency is not actually possible

I know I just said that I like being outside my comfort zone, and that only a few days ago, I said that maybe we don't need to be scared every day.

I take heart from the fact that Nobel Prize–winning psychologist Daniel Kahneman says that it's not possible for us to be completely consistent in our beliefs. In his interview for the *On Being* podcast, he also called the ideal and idea of rationality (which we usually think of as including consistency) as "psychological nonsense."

How refreshing. We are mutable creatures, which means we are capable of more change than we think.

Be inconsistent. Try things on. Change your size. Let your heart get bigger and bigger and . . .

March 22

. . . a heart getting bigger

Here are a couple of things that expand my heart.

I love reading aloud to others and I love being read to. Sometimes, though, the very passage that has assailed my heart is the one I want to read aloud, and I can't make it through, because I'm crying.

Almost every trail-running event I've ever participated in that was longer than two hours brought me to tears at some point—frustration or joy, sometimes both.

March 23

. . . walking

Here's another heart moment.

Today I walked through the park on my way to an appointment, something I rarely do. Usually I'm running or cycling when I'm in there. It was a misty afternoon. I was alone, stone-cold sober, and I got that alternate-reality, trippy feeling of communion with the water-speckled air, the winter-dozing trees, even the siren a few blocks away. The calm elation of being in the right place, my place in the world.

We never know when the world will reach for us; lift its veil to reveal the unspeakable glory of the ordinary.

March 24

. . . don't get bogged down in potential

So much potential (for change, for joy) can be energizing. But what if we take that to its limit. That's where the extreme potentialist flounders.

It's been scientifically shown that if we have too many choices, we are less happy. Too many shampoos are a muddle. So your hair is still dirty. The perfect couch must be out there. In the meantime, you've been sitting on the floor for two years. Choosing in the midst of so much perceived potential becomes a decision that takes too long.

If we are always looking for the next and better possibility, we will never execute, never enjoy the moment, never buy the shampoo, sit on a couch, or get on with the living.

We can take our search for potential too far.

March 25

. . . the pace of life

When the fastest songs come on in my spin class, my legs can't always find the beat right away. When I chase the song, I invariably have trouble meshing with the music. When I close my eyes and let the rhythm come to me, there's a moment when my legs click in and suddenly the beat feels manageable. I know the song isn't actually slower. Yet I feel as if the music has opened up, invited me inside, created space and custom-fitted the rhythm around me.

Sometimes, instead of chasing down potential, we need to let life in.

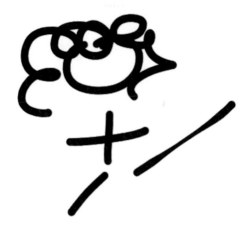

Kick open those doors of opportunity.
Credit: Mina Samuels

March 26

. . . kicking girl

After a long coffee date with a brand-new friend, she walked me to a meeting I had with the executive director of a play incubator (that is—helping new plays find their voice and stage). I had a play in development. I am not very good at such meetings and was bemoaning my insufficiency as we got to the address. My friend pep-talked. Then, just as we were parting, I gave a high kick of absolute ninja-esque confidence.

She laughed. The moment sealed our friendship. I strode in the front door of the midtown Manhattan building.

The kick gave me the juice I needed for the meeting. Though that specific connection has yet to yield fruit, the kick reminded me that, while we do need to be mindful of letting ourselves slip into the rhythms life sends our way, we also need to keep kicking open the doors of opportunity.

March 27

. . . bringing ourselves to our sports

In her 2018 commencement address to the graduating class at Bard, Olympic gold medalist and former soccer player extraordinaire Abby Wambach said: "Soccer didn't make me who I was. I brought who I was to soccer and I get to bring who I am wherever I go. And guess what? So do you."

March 28

. . . with lightness

Our sports remind us that even if the goal, the ambition, the challenge feels serious and heavy, we must bring lightness with us. Forcing an effort might work for a while, but in the end, if we have a long-term relationship with our sports, we know that what will get us out of bed and into our running shorts with the greatest ease is a light heart. Knowing that we take pleasure in our athletic selves is how we find the fun inside the responsibility.

March 29

. . . air barre and pizza

I saw a woman today wearing a T-shirt that read, "My head says air barre, but my heart says pizza."

Why does that have to be a choice? Both, please.

March 30

. . . we are all responsible

Let's take a pause here as we approach the end of the first quarter of the year. Let's step back from reflections about our personal efforts toward strength and balance, to think again about meaning. Why do we do any of what we do?

Rabbi Abraham Joshua Heschel was a great social activist (he was on the front line at Selma with Martin Luther King, Jr.), a mystic, and a twentieth-century religious intellectual. Heschel put it this way: "In a free society, some are guilty, but all are responsible."

Our responsibility is to leave the world a tiny bit better than we found it. Whether it's cleaner bathrooms or showing a girl her strength, we find a way to serve our common humanity.

March 31

... pumping up my tires

In the cold season I abandon my bike in preference to my cross-country skis, and over the winter I let my tires deflate. So when spring comes around, it's time to excavate the bike pump. Some sports I enjoy in the chill and some I don't. Ski and cold go together. I'll run in almost any weather. When I was younger I would bundle up and go out on my bike in weather as cold as 24 degrees Fahrenheit. But at the end I'd be so cold it was as if I was wearing a skin-suit made of ice and no length of hot shower could melt it away. Every year now the minimum temperature at which I'm willing to bike seems to go up a degree or two. My standards are global warming on fast-forward.

For this book, April 1 is my first bike ride. I know that's way late for some of you. We each have our own personal seasonal rhythms. How wonderful.

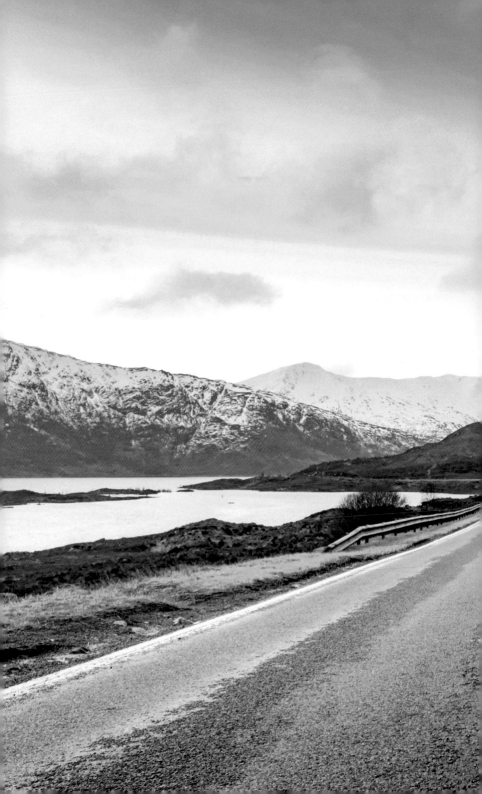

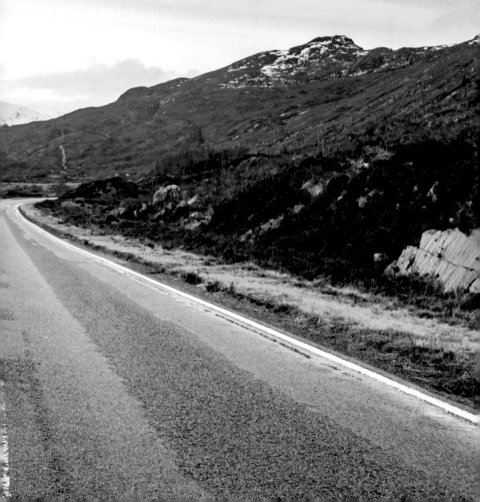

APRIL

April 1

. . . we belong to everything

On this first spring morning, other bikers swarm past me, parting and regrouping like a school of fish. Their shiny, Lycra outfits are mobile billboard advertisements for a host of companies and products. I have no sponsors, no team, nor other affiliations to promote, no one counting on me to be out here representing. I have friends and acquaintances, clients, family, and a cat, but none of them is the least invested in whether I'm actually on my bike this morning, or any other for that matter.

For a moment I feel marooned on my bicycle. Belonging to nothing. Each pedal stroke an exercise in futility. But it's the first warmish morning and I can smell spring. The happy-face daffodils are a-bloom everywhere, with their bright orange centers and frill of butter-yellow petals. The furry buds of magnolias-to-be look like dormant insects on the bare branches and the first hints of pink on the cherry trees glow in the early light.

I'm not nearly alone. I belong to everything.

April 2

. . . kindness

"April is the cruellest month, breeding/ Lilacs out of the dead land, mixing/ Memory and desire, stirring/ Dull roots with spring rain."

In this cruelest month (according to T. S. Eliot), I think about George Saunders's 2013 commencement address at the University of Syracuse. That writer suggested to the class that cultivating kindness was at least as valuable as any career aspirations they might nurture. It's a lesson we all need to take to heart.

April 3

. . . joy in stone

"Write your sorrows in sand and etch your joys in stone," an old Chinese saying goes.

When I'm running, if my mind isn't busy, busy, busy (which is a lot of the time), I think about breathing in joy and breathing out all the thoughts that aren't serving me. I can guarantee myself a good run on the stone foundation of joy.

April 4

. . . loss

Today is my father's birthday. The year before he died, when I called to wish him a happy day, he spent quite some time describing to me, in intimate detail, the ins and outs of airline regulations regarding the size and weight of checked and carry-on baggage. He narrated at length about how he had measured and weighed his, and my mother's, existing luggage, and what new luggage might be necessary to meet the precision of the regulations. We then moved onto the subject of changing out the winter tires for summer tires. And the Canadian Foreign Minister's recent trip to the United Arab Emirates, which involved a visit to a Tim Horton's (Canada's famous donut store, named after a hockey player, of course), and a ride in a silver Mini Cooper.

My mother and I owned Minis at the time. Our cool quotient was elevated.

I thought, *This is ludicrous, why aren't we discussing something more personal, something more important, why aren't we having a deep and honest conversation about what matters in our lives.* We both knew how sick he was.

Then, I thought, I will miss his singularity when he's gone. So I kept listening

I was right—I do miss it.

April 5

. . . nostalgia

My partner thinks I was born without a nostalgia gene, because I'm not generally attached to the *things* imbued with memories, like pinecone-skier Christmas tree ornaments. Yet, I write to explore and re-explore, to transform the past into story, to find where we belong inside that story. I write about women and sports, because I want to understand the transformative impact I felt in my own life. To add my own drop of kindling to the fire strong women bring to the world.

I am nostalgic for the stories.

April 6

...glow

A storm was coming and I was driving. The light on the mountains was like black light in nightclubs, which makes everything that's white glow—clothes, teeth, the whites of eyes. The window glass of houses on the hillside glowed against the muted green-silver essence of the trees.

I almost drove off the road trying to email myself a description of what I'd seen. I wanted so much to tell you about it. There's no obscure sports message in this day. It's just a nostalgia pause for natural beauty

April 7

...thoughts on skirts

When I sit down, the skirt waistband ends up around my armpits, and when I walk the skirt spins around. I can't wear this seemingly innocuous, ubiquitous article of clothing. To get a skirt over my hips means that I'll be swimming inside the waistband, which can set off insecurities about my body shape. Mostly I stick to dresses.

Until running skirts, that is. With them, it was love at first run. In the warmer months now, I'm almost monogamous with running skirts. I have two neglected pairs of shorts, for when the laundry just isn't getting done.

You'll notice I said love at first *run* and not *sight*. That's because the prissy feminist in me initially resisted the fashion as insufficiently strong and independent. Until I wore it and discovered the psychological retro-rockets hidden beneath the skirt. Strong. Capable. Powerful. And yes . . . sexy.

Run like a girl!

April 8

. . . running skirts at memorials

I was staying in an apartment on Ile de la Cite in Paris, around the corner from Notre Dame, for a couple of months one year. Our regular run was along the Seine. Sometimes we would stretch in the gardens behind the cathedral, but one day my partner and I thought maybe we'd finish with a stretch in the gardens of the Deportation Museum across from the church garden. We hadn't gone into the garden or memorial. It was only as we went through the gate that we realized the garden wasn't open to the public, unless we had tickets to the memorial. *Why not?* We bought tickets.

Then the security guard motioned me over to discuss my attire. My skirt, she said, was too short. I was mortified and felt horribly rude about the inappropriateness of my outfit. Perhaps sensing my remorse, she relented. Once inside, I was conscious of the need to hold my body in an extra-respectful position. The memorial was overwhelming in its simplicity. On the way out, I stopped in the garden and sat on a bench to absorb what I'd seen. The security guard headed in my direction. *Oh no.*

"How was it?" she asked.

"It was moving," I said.

"It is," she said. And then, "Have a nice day."

I sat up straighter, pressing my bare knees together.

April 9

... flying and flocking

Riding Citibike to one of my yoga studios takes me across 40th Street from the Hudson River bike path. Fortieth Street is all about the Lincoln Tunnel, connecting New Jersey to Manhattan beneath the Hudson River. In high-traffic hours it's a mess of large trucks, buses, and cars driven by people who still think leaning on their horns accomplishes something. Plus, as a result of all that heavy traffic, the road is grooved and pitted.

At Dyer Avenue, there's a curlicue of overhead roads. All those girders with ledges protected from the elements attract the pigeons. No, this is not about getting crapped on. Because, though the birds do a lot of sitting and cooing, what they seem to do most is flock and fly. They make big circles above the road, dipping and swooping. I crane my neck as I wait for the light to change. Traffic thunders past me, only inches away. The road is sooty and greasy. Flattened plastic bottles crunch under my bike tires. But above, through the curled-lattice of roads, are sky and cloud and birds on the wing. Light. Free. When I look up, I feel that, too.

Green light. I plunge back into the *swoosh* of metal and

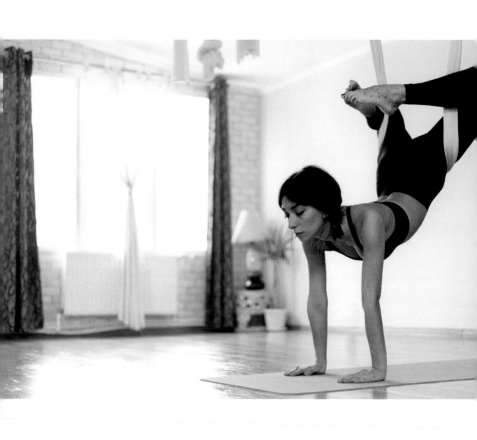

wheels. I carry the float of the birds with me. I'm going to fly, too, on a hammock at aerial yoga.

April 10

. . . the pursuit of alignment

When Christopher Harrison, the founder of Anti-Gravity Lab who developed a broad range of aerial yoga techniques, needed guinea pigs for a new healing massage and stretch protocol he was developing, I offered myself up. I'm always game to experiment with different physical wellness modalities— acupuncture, cupping, dry needling, chiropractic, deep tissue massage, structural integration, to name a few. I can tolerate a reasonable amount of pain in the pursuit of alignment.

For more than two hours, my body was stretched and manipulated. Sore points discovered and pressured. There were brief moments of pleasure, but for the most part it was an experience of wild pain. I hoped it would manifest benefits after I left. It did and sooner than I expected.

April 11

. . . riding no-handed

Riding the bike home after two painful hours of manipulation, I was gentle with myself. I kept the bike geared lower than usual and let the pedals spin. I felt a full body ease and alignment. A thought floated into my consciousness: "I'm going to ride no-handed."

I am very comfortable on a bicycle. I ride around the city. I ride on roads and trails. But I never ride without at least one hand on the handlebars. I've always envied those who can ride no-handed. I tried.

Just like that I was skimming the world, pedals flowing out of the soles of my feet, rooted lightly to the bicycle seat. As happy as can be.

Was I more aligned physically? Was I more open to trying? Both. Opening space in our bodies can open space in our minds, if we are willing to let our minds and bodies have the conversation.

April 12

. . . air barre rapture

Doing Anti-Gravity air barre one Easter weekend, I was struck by the ritual elements. We were doing deep twists, expelling toxins. As if last night's wine were being wrung out of us like a confession. The pain of the effort was our rapture.

April 13

. . . self-compassion

Forget last night's wine. The biggest toxin we need to expel with our twisting is self-criticism. Forgiving ourselves is the most important detox.

Here's an approach:

Step one—form the intention to be easier on yourself, to judge yourself less harshly, to have compassion for your own mistakes.

Step two—notice the self-talk cluttering your mind. When is it harsh? Why? No surprise, meditation is one of the best ways to make a practice of noticing.

Step three—when you notice self-criticism, talk to yourself with the same kindness you would extend to a child or a friend. Kindness is not leniency. Kindness is not, "so what you made a mistake, it doesn't matter." No. Kindness knows that we all make mistakes, that we are doing our best, and that a mistake does not mean we are worthless or lazy or a bad person.

Step four—notice how kindness feels. Our brain is wired to reinforce behavior that is rewarded with pleasure. Instead of saying to yourself, you suck, because you cut your run short; say—great job that you got out there on a tough day!

Step five—forgive yourself if you don't always notice.

April 14

... rolling out our heart muscle

As I was rolling out my IT band this morning (cue suppressed screams of agony), I thought to myself: *The heart is a muscle.* What would a roller for the heart muscle look like? What if we could literally roll out the knots in our heart, the blockages and the closed and clenched bits? Can you imagine how painful it would be to tenderize all those lumps of hurt and hate and fear? And yet, how gorgeous your heart would feel afterward?

April 15

... our tenderized hearts

When we tenderize our heart muscle, we become more vulnerable. That's hard. Have you ever sworn off relationships or having a pet, because you just don't want to face another loss? To forswear loss is to hide from love's light.

Louise Glück writes in her poem, "Fable," "But the light will give us no peace."

Indeed. Love's light is not serene. Love is a raging fire, a foaming river and a precipitous cliff that demands that we accept loss. As poet and philosopher David Whyte puts it, "Will you become a full citizen of vulnerability?"

Can we keep opening and accepting in the face of what we will bear witness to under the bright light of love?

April 16

. . . tenderizing is a process

We don't just roll out our IT bands (or hamstrings, or shins, or lower backs) once and we're done. Likely we have to keep at the project of breaking down the inflamed pretzels of our muscles, which resist efforts to smooth them out.

The pain of rolling is always worth it in the end. It's a thing we can only learn by persisting. So it is with our hearts. It takes all our strength to keep rolling out our hearts.

April 17

. . . the courage of the light

"The greatest courage is to keep our eyes open to the light, as on death."

—Albert Camus

April 18

. . . let go of blame

Perhaps the most difficult challenge in rolling out our hearts is letting go of our intense need to ascribe blame. Even if we are blaming ourselves, we want somebody to be at fault, as if fault explains the chaos that is the world.

Yet, if we scrape away the surface of blame, we will always unearth another layer of blame, and another.

When we are busy finding someone to blame (even if that someone is ourselves), our attention is diverted from the real work. With blame out of the picture, we are left with our power (and responsibility!) to learn from our mistakes and to make better choices.

April 19

. . . perfection

How can we attain the indefinable? Why would we set an unreachable goal? Making the impossible possible is more likely. Some people say every moment of our lives is perfect for that moment. I hear that intellectually, but I can't help thinking: "Yes, but some moments are more perfect." The moment I broke my foot, for example, was at the low end of the perfect scale.

Our sports show us that our best is not about some nebulous idea of perfection, but about the heart we bring to our effort that day.

April 20

. . . moving our emotions through the bloodstream

In times when I'm a hot mess (example: crying uncontrollably in the Times Square subway station because the train I need is out of service, but obviously something else is bothering me too and I just can't figure out what), the world feels quite a few light years away from perfect. I take refuge in my runs, my rides, my yoga hammock, or whatever the season's activity is. Those days will never be my best workouts (even if they are perfect for that day). But they allow my emotions to move through the currents of my bloodstream, so the fog can lift, even if it's just a little.

April 21

. . . accepting uncertainty

On a World Science Festival panel that I attended, neuroscientist Lisa Barrett argued that our brains seek out certainty to lower the stress level in our bodies. Stress uses metabolic energy in our system, so the less stressed we are, the more energy we have available in our "body budget," as she called it. The more time we have to spend on more fruitful activities than stressing out.

But certainty is a mirage. Life can change in less than a heartbeat. How can we de-stress?

Zoran Josipovic, another neuroscientist on the same panel, researches nonduality. He studies the brains of experienced meditators, like Buddhist monks. No, meditation doesn't help us obtain certainty, he says. Rather it teaches us to accept uncertainty.

We feel this truth in our sports. While I use my sports to de-stress on days that I'm feeling overwhelmed, my best workouts happen when my mind is not hanging on tightly to what's wrong and instead is open and pliable. The ability to accept and thrive in uncertainty is just another way to describe the flow we all have access to, if we are willing to ease off the accelerator and brakes, to let go.

Meditation can be part of our workout regime. Our workouts can be moving meditations.

April 22

. . . OM

I love the sound of rolling *OM*s that happens when the whole yoga class chants *OM* over and over again, everyone in her own time, at her own pitch. After the first *OM*, the sounds begin to move apart, until the sound of *OM* rolls over itself in a wave pattern, sometimes cresting together, sometimes lulling together, sometimes crossing, a sound that is like the ocean, like my own blood pumping in my ears. It is a sound that lifts me out of myself, a sound that contains and expresses the harmony that exists at the core of our chaotic-seeming universe. It is a sound that calms and invigorates my body, joining my physical and emotional self.

April 23

. . . superstitious attachment

I engage in my fair share of superstitious behaviors. There are topics I don't like to comment on out loud or even think about, because I think I'll jinx the outcome. Don't say there's no traffic, because the two-hour delay in a snarl of cars is just ahead. Don't point out that you are going through an injury-free period, because plantar fasciitis can hear you. Don't brag about your job security.

I used to think that my superstition was a version of the Buddhist concept of non-attachment. Although we may enjoy something enormously in the moment, we ought not to become attached to the object of our enjoyment, so that we depend on it for our inner fulfillment.

But my superstition is its own form of attachment. It's just another form of worrying about whether something is going to be taken away.

We should revel in all that is good in our lives. Notice the joy of a comfortable run. Allow the feeling to soak in. Let go of expectation.

April 24

. . . small gifts

All those small moments of joy are gifts, not to be hoarded or covered in plastic in some vain effort to preserve their freshness. No. They are to be savored right now, in all their fullness.

Take a few seconds at the end of every workout to think about how you felt. Pick out in particular the bits where you felt good. While there is no formaldehyde preservative for our memories, to note them specifically is a fine place to start. To ensure that when we store them away in the file drawers of our memory banks, we have distilled their richest flavor. We have access to their essence, not to hang on to, but to refresh our gratitude in the moments it might be running low.

April 25

. . . reliable friends

Friendship is an implicit contract of sorts. We promise to show up for our friends.

Different periods of my life are bookmarked by who my running or cycling mates were at the time, or who joined me at yoga. I take great pleasure in scrolling through the images of all those hours of focused company, the conversations, the gift of their reliability.

April 26

... absent friends

Right next to the pleasure of recalling all the friends I've sported with over the years is the gentle hint of sadness at their current absence. With each person there is a particular spot along one of our routes that will evoke them. For many years a friend and I used to run the "loop plus a loop," as we called it. That is—the loop of Central Park, plus a loop of the reservoir in the middle of the park. She is with me now every time I run on the reservoir path. Hill repeats on the north hill in Central Park reunites a disparate gathering of mates. A series of friends who have drifted away accompany me any time I ride up to Nyack, joining me at different points

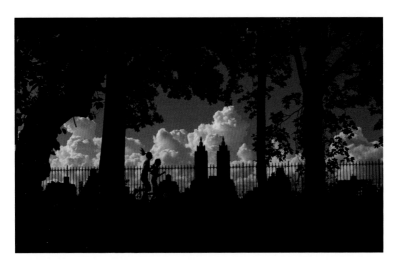

Two women running on the Central Park Reservoir. *Credit: Mark Gurevich*

along the route—as I cross the George Washington Bridge, as I climb out of Palisades Park on the long hill up to the ranger station, or as I deke through Tallman State Park.

Even when we are working out alone, our absent friends accompany us on the roads and trails.

April 27

. . . pink clothing

I am pink. My skin looks like the shade of the inside of an Easter bunny's ear. If I wear pink, I disappear inside my clothes, like a creature turned inside out.

Okay, it's more than that. I feel weak in pink. Helpless. Fragile. Delicate. Frail. Limp. Insignificant. Less than.

I feel just the right amount of tough when I'm wearing my favorite clothing color—black.

Except when I am doing a sport. Then, I've been known to rock an eye-popping pink here and there. With a little mud and sweat, there's no room for fragile.

April 28

. . . floating cherry-blossom petals

The cherry-blossom petals are beautiful in spring, as they

float through the air, landing in my hair like confetti. Until I inhale one and start coughing.

There's something sticky on the petals (is it the ambient spring pollen?) that lodges them firmly in my throat. Tenacious and not half as delicate as they appear—just like little girls.

April 29

. . . parkour birthday parties for girls

I was working at a table in the coffee shop this morning and beside me four mothers were having a conversation about birthday parties. One said that her daughter wanted to have a sports party. Specifically a parkour party, that urban obstacle course sport that entails moving as fast as possible through the environment while running, jumping, climbing, and such. (I'm not sure how a parkour birthday party works, but can I come?)

The mother in question was concerned. Apparently girls don't generally like sports and thus it would be hard to make the party palatable for her daughter's friends.

Title IX, legislation ensuring equal opportunity in sports for girls and women, was implemented in the seventies. This is how far we have come in forty years. When we get out there for our run, or our ride, or our rugby game, or whatever the sport is that calls us, we are not doing it only for ourselves, but as an example for all the girls who want parkour birthday parties.

April 30

. . . why can't women figure skaters wear pants?

Rachel, the former figure skater we met back in February, has a daughter who would likely be very excited by a parkour birthday party. Rachel's six-year-old has asked her more than once why the women figure skaters have to wear skirts. She has declared that she has no interest in pursuing her mother's teen sport unless she can wear pants, pointing out that ice rinks are cold and it must hurt more to fall without pants on.

A wise-beyond-her-years and ferocious girl, I'm angling for an invite to her future birthday parties.

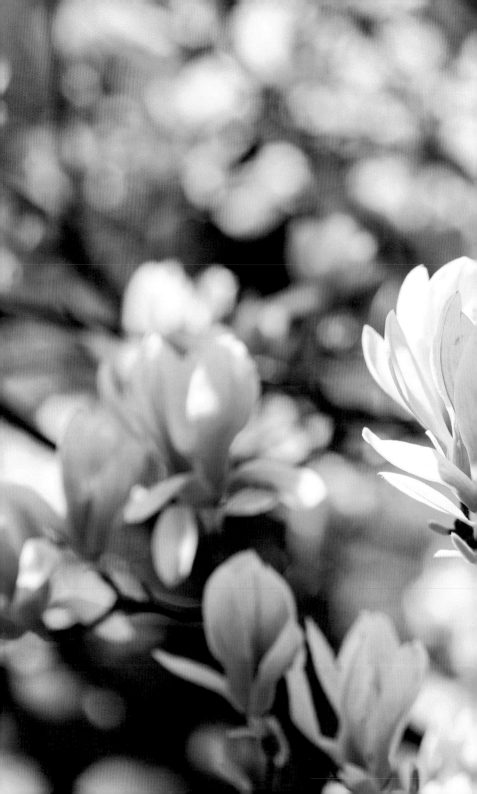

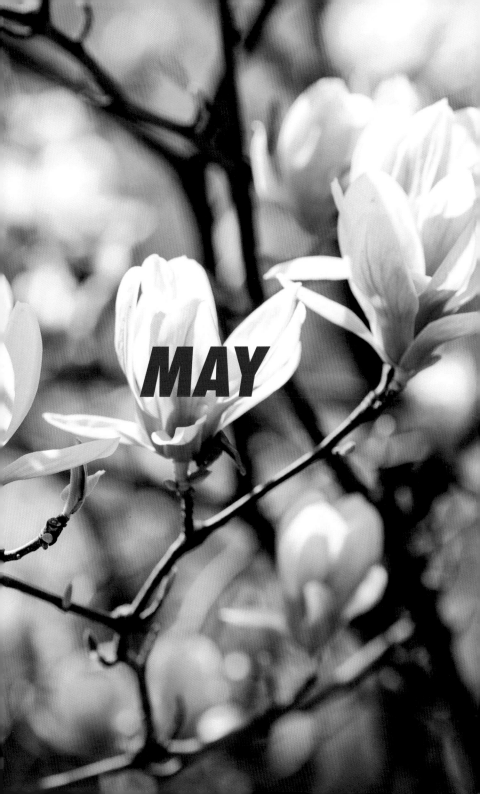

MAY

May 1

... Notorious RBG

In the opening moments of the documentary *RBG* about Ruth Bader Ginsburg, the eighty-three-year-old Supreme Court Justice is holding plank position as her trainer counts down slowly from twenty-five, occasionally making adjustments to her posture. Not only has RBG made an enormous

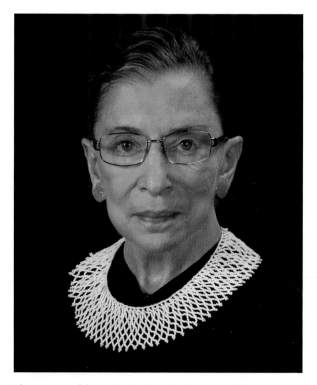

The Honorable Ruth Bader Ginsburg's official SCOTUS portrait.

contribution to the women's rights movement, she is keeping herself strong, so that she can continue to serve us on the High Court for as long as possible. Her voice makes a difference, whether she is with the majority or dissenting. We are beneficiaries of RBG's time in the gym.

May 2
. . . putting in the work

"I'm a consistent person. Putting in the work is my achievement. I don't let myself quit," says Auditi, who works as a senior vice president at a national education organization. As with RBG, we all benefit from Auditi's work of ensuring our children get great learning opportunities. When it comes to her workouts, Auditi plans ahead and measures her constancy. That said, Auditi listens when her body tells her she needs to change things up from too much running, or take an extra day of rest.

She brings this same discipline and listening into her work. While she strives to be her best at work and expects the same of others, she knows that standard has to be balanced with humanity.

May 3

. . . a differentiator

Auditi is, like many women (including me), an adult-onset athlete. Early in life, she was focused on being smart, singing, playing the clarinet and other school-related activities. It wasn't until university that she found running and began to define herself as an athlete. There's that word again. Athlete sounds daunting, but it's time we women owned that word more.

Auditi still remembers the first time she had a conversation with a group of coworkers, also athletes. They pulled a thread between the demands of their athletics and how that consistency enabled them to perform better in their work. They all felt that being an athlete was a differentiator in their career. Her career may be about helping minds develop, but she knows how implicated the body is in that process.

Her sports are a place she practices discipline. Her sports ground her, especially when work is ultra-busy. Her sports are a constant companion, when she's traveling all over the place. And, of course, when stress levels run high, her sports are a place to reset and take a new breath.

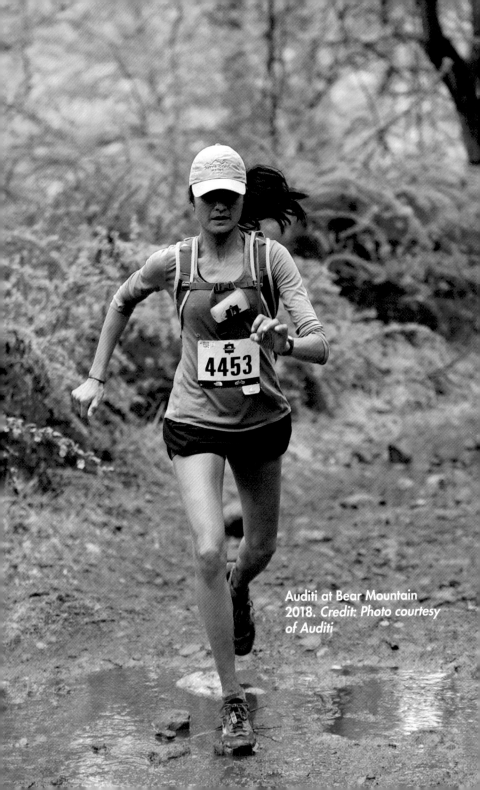

Auditi at Bear Mountain 2018. Credit: Photo courtesy of Auditi

May 4

. . . leave the princesses in our dust

The princess effect is sucking the life out of girls, leaving them on the front stoop, waiting for Prince Charming, instead of outside running around in the fresh air, where they might not look pretty-in-pink every moment and their tiara might fall off. The Women's Sports Foundation reports that girls drop out of sports at a rate of 6:1 versus boys. And a Girl Scout study showed that many girls between eleven and seventeen years old don't play sports because they think their bodies don't look good. When I watched the movie *Frozen*, I was struck by Elsa's transformation, which included high heels, a classic wasp waist, and more cleavage than I can produce, even with a lot of padding.

We cannot let the girls in our lives grow up like this. The world needs women's strength, women like RBG, all the women in this book, and you!

May 5

. . . our bodies are meant for sports

Even if girls do think their bodies look good, there are a lot of messages out there that we shouldn't be using our bodies for sports. Passing through Times Square subway station one day,

I was struck by a particularly troubling Levi's ad. The boys in it were skateboarding and doing tricks on bikes wearing their jeans. The one girl in the ad had her jeans down around her ankles (she's ostensibly pulling them on, after what, who knows, since she's standing beside an SUV in the middle of nowhere with several boys), flashing us a good look at her lace panties. The tagline is about creating our legacy.

So . . . boys' legacies lie in extreme sports and girls' legacies in their frilly undergarments and taking off their pants.

We know better than that. Let's pass it on.

May 6

. . . the wrong socks

The rain stopped a few minutes before we started the half marathon, a run on the trails around Bear Mountain, hilly and technical. I had trained adequately, but not spectacularly. I was wearing the wrong socks, thin ones meant for road running. I was in my trail runners. Two years earlier, the last time I'd done this same event, I'd won my age group and performed well overall among women. This time I felt like the only question was how much worse my performance would be. Forget the socks. My head was in the wrong place. This was not going to be a legacy day. What happened next was hardly a surprise.

May 7

... not the best trail half marathon

I hadn't run 100 meters in the half marathon before I knew
it wasn't going to be my day in my body either. My left hamstring zoomed up to level eleven on the ineffectiveness scale. I
was running on one concrete leg. It was an ancient injury, for
which I had recently started some belated acupuncture. The
protocol had opened new access to the strength and flexibility
of my hamstring, but as a result, the muscles were in shock.
As if to say, *WTF, you want us to do our share now?* For
many years those muscles had hidden out, letting my right leg
figure out all sorts of minute ways to take over the work of
the left hamstring.

While my left hamstring eased after a mile, I couldn't find
my mojo and one inner voice was scolding me for my weakness, while the other tried to say soothing things. Hey, that
I could even *hear* that second voice was progress. In an earlier part of my life, the voice of kindness was on mute. Here
she was, not as dominating as I might have hoped, but still
making her points. Which were these: *It's only a race; keep
going; you can push yourself a tiny bit harder; maybe next
time you'll train more precisely; in the meantime, wow, you're
amazing to be out here at all.*

In the end, I was nine minutes slower than two years earlier. I came second in my age group.

Rock star!

May 8

. . . my partner beat me

Yesterday there was a bit of the story I didn't tell you. My partner beat me. I had trained faster and more miles, but he had a phenomenal race. He's strong that way. I envy him. It makes me mad sometimes.

When he passed me on the course, I had a surge of . . . defeat. I wanted to sit down in the muddy leaves on the side of the trail—ticks be damned—and just give up. I wanted to holler about unfairness. Instead I let the kind voice talk me on. After all, I was in the middle of the woods, and there didn't seem any way other way to get to the end.

He was waiting for me at the finish line with a big smile and open arms. When I saw him like that, I knew what a risk he had taken. I might have sulk-run past him, pushed him away and generally behaved like a child. I had done that before. He chose to believe in my capacity to get over myself.

I did not disappoint him.

May 9

. . . Orange Theory

A friend emailed me her Orange Theory workout results, to show me the detailed statistics that are tracked around her performance in each class, comparing her over time and against other participants. Orange Theory, in case you haven't heard, is yet another version of a boot-camp workout.

Seeing her stats made me question the balance I'd struck between statistics and how-I-feel (aka instinct and intuition). When I first started racing, I spent a decent amount of time looking at my watch and tracking various results. I never got into the heart-rate monitor though, and then, after about fifteen years, I stopped racing. I switched my focus from road running races and triathlons to "events" like long trail runs and ultra marathons. I derive most of my motivation from the pleasures and rewards of staying active and healthy, fit and strong.

Now I've gotten to the point where I basically never measure or track anything I do (except after the fact—I know, I know, that's exactly when all I'm doing is comparing). Yes, I am conscious of how many days I work out a week (almost always six) and I try to push hard in some undefined proportion of those workouts and take it easier in another undefined portion. In the balance of going with how I feel, versus what the stats say, I am operating only on the first and not using the statistics at all to guide me.

May 10

... what am I capable of?

Without statistics, I don't know what more I might be capable of. I am sure that I'm capable of more than what I did at the trail half marathon (after all, only two years earlier I had run nine minutes faster under similar conditions).

The question is, what do I want to be capable of, and what else is on my *what-am-I-capable-of* plate?

Athletics is only one small piece of my life. My sports are about supporting the rest of my life, not dictating the terms. Yet writing this book, by its very nature, demands that my sports remain a priority. To find that balance, where the equilibrium between my sports and my life are just so, that is an ongoing exploration. At the moment, instinct runs the show for my athletics. But that's not to say that statistics might not get the upper hand another day.

May 11

. . . orthodoxy in workouts and elsewhere

At meditation, the teacher for the evening gave a talk that seemed to meander through all the different traditions of Buddhism, as well as examples of people he knew who were intermingling different versions of Christianity or Judaism or Islam with their Buddhism. At first, I couldn't quite follow the point of his string of random stories about unorthodox approaches to meditation. Then I realized that the very structure of his talk, its loose nature and its open-ended flow, *was* the point.

Orthodoxy, in any form, is constrictive and can lead to violence, whether that violence is physical or mental. Because when we adhere to one point of view too strongly, we are likely to force our beliefs on another (or ourselves) in a way contrary to human flourishing.

There's always a new sport or class that's being touted

as the "only workout you'll ever need." That's orthodoxy. What we need is to listen to our body. How does it like the workout? Are there any violent results—injury, lack of sleep, physical depletion? Do we feel healthy and strong? Our body changes, too. It's not a one-time check-in.

Experiment. Consider the results. Adjust what doesn't work. Improve what works. Repeat.

Listen. Open. Soften.

May 12

. . . quitting can be strategic

A heretic is a person who holds controversial opinions, especially one who publicly dissents from the officially accepted dogma. Avoiding orthodoxy can feel heretical. It also means you are thinking for yourself; gathering facts, listening, drawing conclusions.

While nobody wants to be a quitter, sometimes quitting is the exact thing that needs to be done. One of the things Elizabeth learned from rugby, that she carried with her into running a forty-million-dollar company, was that focusing on competitive advantages necessitates letting go of things we don't do well or that don't suit us.

May 13

. . . what's right for you

Just because *everybody* is doing high-intensity interval training, or boxing, or long slow distance, doesn't mean it's right for you. The only way you can figure out what sports your body loves and responds to is to try them on. See how an athletic pursuit fits. And quit when it's not right for you.

I pursued aerial arts for about a year. I learned how to climb a *silk*, wind myself up in the strong, stretchy fabric that hangs from high rafters, then flip and spin my way out. One day, just as I was starting to feel comfortable in the practice, I almost ripped my arm off grabbing at the silk in a moment of fear. Once my shoulder healed, I started back at the practice, but my heart wasn't in it anymore. I kept forcing myself to go, because I thought, *Well I've already invested a year on a steep learning curve. I can't quit now.* Yet I'd known, even before the injury, that I would never make the time to become as good as I'd like. I would have had to give up other sports I loved (such as running), not to mention that after the shoulder incident I better understood that I risked an injury, which could sideline my true passions.

Still, I'm glad I tried. The experience of learning something radically different from anything I had ever done before was mind-bending.

But I'm glad I quit. Soon after I was introduced to aerial yoga, which fulfilled my craving to fly.

May 14

. . . just quit and just do it

At forty-two, Kimberly had a high-paying, prestigious job and financial security. She was living what we might call *the good life* in America. Then she realized that what she had was not what she wanted. She made a list of things that were important to her: to travel; to do something that helped people; to give back to the world in a meaningful way; and to incorporate her love of cycling into that mix of travel and purpose.

Around the same time, Kimberly learned about Project Rwanda, a non-profit that designed and distributed special cargo bikes for coffee (one of Rwanda's key crops) at low cost. Six months later, she was on a plane to Rwanda for a three-month volunteer stint, which turned into paid work, which led to her involvement with Team Rwanda, the national cycling team, and getting in the best cycling shape of her life, and eight years in Rwanda on a shoestring budget.

She's back in Wyoming now, living an active life, close to the land. Early in the Rwanda experience, when asked how she made the move, Kimberly said, "The secret of how I did it is . . . I quit."

While we may not be ready to give up our lives and move to Africa, Kimberly reminds us to think: *What can I do more of? What can I do with less of?*

May 15

. . . the obstacles are part of our dreams

Here's another way to think about the strategic value of quitting. We've all likely heard by now about positive thinking. The idea that if we just go after something with enough intention, then our dream will come true. Well, new research into the science of motivation suggests that it's not that straightforward. That, in fact, we may need to disengage from wishes that are unfeasible, to focus on those that are possible.

Gabriele Oettingen, professor of psychology at NYU and author of *Rethinking Positive Thinking: Inside the New Science of Motivation*, writes that when we are listing our goals and dreams, it is crucial to list the obstacles too. If we envision the obstacles as much as the dreams and goals, then we are more likely to succeed. Her particular technique is called WOOP—wish, outcome, obstacle, plan.

What is your dream? What will life look like if you fulfill your dream? What obstacles inside of you stand in your way?

Make a plan to address those obstacles.

May 16

. . . focus on the obstacles inside

Notice that the obstacles Gabriele asks people to focus on are those inside. For example, while I was writing this book, the task at hand, the wish, was to sit down at my desk and write. The desired outcome was weekly progress. While I love writing, a book is daunting. The siren song of procrastination can be very loud indeed. All manner of other tasks can subvert my intention to write, and I can even justify them under the heading of research for the book. Another challenge is turning off my internal editor and critic, who can make writing impossible. Not to mention the imposter syndrome, a plague that afflicts too many women.

These are some of the obstacles inside of me—I overcome them by setting daily or weekly writing goals, which do not require publication-ready writing, but just words on the page, to be edited later.

But other obstacles, those outside of me, are not as easily surmounted. And that's where Gabriele makes it clear that we need to let go of the wishes that distract us. Only then can we give our attention to the dreams we can fulfill.

May 17

. . . the fallacy of sunk costs

One of the great challenges in letting go of a dream—or anything in which you've invested time or money—is the notion that we've put resources toward the dream already: how can we give up on it? Instead, we keep sinking more resources into a losing project, hoping to somehow resuscitate it—whether it's a relationship, a job, or tickets for a trip we don't want to take. That's the fallacy of sunk costs in operation.

We may have trained hard for a marathon, but in the last week we are plagued by shin pain. If we lay off now, then we can avoid the looming stress fracture. But, oh, that marathon we've trained hard for is calling out to us. Is it worth all the time off afterward to heal the injury?

I could never answer that question for you. The important thing is that we ask ourselves the right questions, that we are honest about the obstacles and feasibility of our dreams. When you know what's worth fighting for—go for it with all your heart.

May 18

. . . goals vs. habits

As supportive as habits can be, they are one of the things that can lead us into the fallacy of sunk costs. Habits are wonderful—brushing our teeth, saying thank you, getting our butts out of bed for a workout. But when we rely on them too heavily, they can create a bias toward themselves. That is, having a lot of habits can lead us to use habit as our action-strategy. But habitual action-strategies may cause us to lose our goal orientation—addictions, for example, are an extreme manifestation of relying too much on a habit.

So we need to have habits and goals, two separate psychological motivators. Scientific studies are literally locating the different synaptic transactions in our brain, which govern the balance between goal-directed and habitual action. Of course, part of the aim of such research is to find the chemical stimulants or repressors, which might be used to cause us to either build a habit or break a habit.

In the meantime, it's still on us to assess where a habit will help us, and where the focus of a particular goal serves us better. As with everything, the key is balance. Have I said that before? *Yes!* Will I say it again? *Yes!*

The current energy that animates all that we are and aspire to be is the constant dynamic tension of finding, maintaining, losing, and finding balance.

May 19

. . . gratefulness + thanksgiving = gratitude

Brother David Steindl-Rast, an Austrian monk and long-time proponent of dialogue between Christian and Buddhist monks, proposes that gratitude is composed of two distinct ingredients: gratefulness, which is the subconscious feeling of joy that wells up in us; and thanksgiving, which is the experience of allowing our gratefulness to overflow and become conscious, to break into thanksgiving, to sing, to dance, to implicate our whole bodies in the feeling and expression of joy. When put together, gratefulness and thanksgiving create gratitude.

But if we cut off our gratefulness instead of letting it overflow, either because something outside ourselves suggests that what we're grateful for is not worthy—not big enough, not expensive enough, not hip enough, or not going to generate enough status—then we do not allow the overflow into the physical sensations of thanksgiving, and thus we don't experience the full power of gratitude.

As Steindl-Rast points out, we can't be grateful for everything in our lives, but we can be grateful every moment. That takes a lot of practice. I'm not there yet.

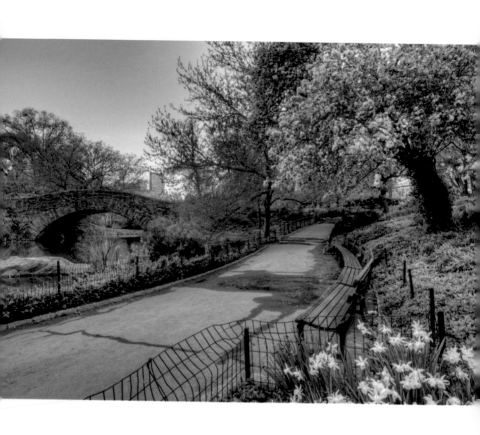

May 20

. . . running grateful

I was running, listening to one of my favorite interview podcasts, when I first heard Brother David Steindl-Rast talk about his definition of gratitude. As his voice soothed through my earbuds, the voice in my head tried to shout him down. The heat that day was debilitating. Even now (months later), I want to say the heat wasn't enough to justify my exhaustion. A part of me is still unforgiving of my slow pace. Meanwhile, Brother David talked about stopping to notice what we are grateful for, instead of running from one thing to the next all the time. He didn't literally mean running, but since I was, I stopped.

I was on a little bridge in Central Park. Obeying the benevolent voice in my ear bud, I walked across slowly, willing myself to be grateful for my health.

Then I heard a violin playing, the sound reverberating under the bridge. I felt like it was my personal musical accompaniment for my grateful moment. I looked underneath the bridge and all around, but I couldn't see the violinist. I'm sure the person was somewhere, or was she? The invisibility of the musician added to the feeling of thanksgiving that overflowed through my body.

I'd like to say that the rest of my run went better. It didn't. Except this—I felt lighter for having given myself the pause.

May 21

... Stop. Look. Go.

So how do we practice Brother David's equation for gratitude? In his writing, he gives us three steps—stop, look, go—which he also codes as awake, aware, alert.

We need to be awake to the world, so we can notice the moments to pause, to stop and be consciously grateful. When are those moments? Anytime. All the time. He describes them as the moments of surprise, even the smallest. The trick is that we need to allow ourselves to be surprised. Oh, but there's nothing really surprising in most of my days, we might think. No? As Brother David points out, "Isn't it surprising that there is anything at all, rather than nothing?" Indeed. We always have something to be grateful for, if we stop.

Then we have to look, to be aware of our surroundings, of the opportunity for joy in circumstances in which we find ourselves, for the people in our lives, for our body, for our mind.

Finally, we need to go with the opportunity. This may be the hardest part, to be alert to the potential for enjoyment within the surprise. Yes, some days we will have to push ourselves a little to go with the joy, but like all practice, this becomes easier over time.

I had to make myself stop during my run. But when the music started, I was transported by the surprise.

May 22

. . . redefining success

How do we define success? What does it mean to each of us to be successful? We each need to define our own idea of success.

Whenever we do an athletic event together, my partner will declare success as soon as we get to the starting line. I know that he's right, but I have a hard time defining that as a success for me. What is it that I need to prove to myself, or is it to others?—That I am worthy.

It is easy to look at every one of you and say, "You are worthy!"

How do I know that for myself?

When we feel worthy, it is because we have allowed ourselves to feel joy and love. Nothing else can give us such a sense of worth.

So I circle back to gratitude and find my worth in the surprise of life, the gift of an invisible violin player on a hot summer run.

May 23

. . . you can do anything, if you can get over your low self-esteem

What a world we live in. We are simultaneously told we can do anything, and yet low self-esteem plagues our society. If you think that's not true, spend some time in the self-help section of a bookstore. There are shelves of books that assure us that if we just think highly enough about ourselves, then everything is possible.

Why is this?

Because if we are told we can do anything, when it turns out not to be true, then our self-esteem has to wrestle with that so-called failure. So writer and philosopher Alain de Botton points out with kindness and wit in his TED talk, *A Kinder, Gentler Philosophy of Success.*

How do we define success? We succeed when our self-worth feels evident. Nothing more. Nothing less. I deserve to be at this starting line, as my partner might say. I showed up, when there are always a million reasons not to. Whatever happens next is up to hazard and randomness. Bring it on—and be grateful for the chance to get to the starting line.

May 24

. . . cultivate a growth mindset

Once we redefine success, so that we know that what we're going for is truly ours, and we've identified not only our wishes, but the very real obstacles, how do we proceed?

With a growth mindset.

In her book, *Mindset: The New Psychology of Success*, Carol Dweck explores the difference between approaching our life with a fixed mindset versus a growth mindset.

In a fixed mindset, we assume that our intelligence, creativity, and ultimately our character are fixed assets, which we can't change in any way. Success is an affirmation of these assets, and failure an assault, one to be avoided at all costs. The fixed mindset, as you can well imagine, does not want us to do anything new, and certainly not anything at which we might fail, especially publicly.

The growth mindset, on the other hand, thrives on challenge and sees failure as a learning opportunity, a chance to improve, to reach higher still. The growth mindset knows (and I say know, because I believe this with all my heart) that we all have the ability to develop and grow; that with hard work and the willingness to get out there and accumulate experience, we may all find new ways of being hidden inside ourselves.

May 25

. . . our unknowable potential

"Do people with this [growth] mindset believe that anyone can be anything, that anyone with proper motivation or education can become Einstein or Beethoven? No," writes Carol Dweck. "But they believe that a person's true potential is unknown (and unknowable); that it's impossible to foresee what can be accomplished with years of passion, toil, and training."

How rejuvenating!

Sounds familiar, too, doesn't it? Because every avenue and side trail we run down, we always come back to balance. It's finding the middle way between our passion, toil, and training, and then letting go of that prevalent platitude that *we can do anything*. It's letting go of the dreams that don't serve us, so the dreams we can grow with have room to flourish.

May 26

. . . learn, learning, never learned

This growth mindset is all about challenging ourselves to learn more. When we are in learning mode, we can't help but grow. When we think we've learned it all—that life is fixed— then our primary hunger for learning is replaced by a hunger for approval. We set aside our efforts to develop ourselves in favor of pursuits that validate us.

Why risk running a marathon, when you've got the 10K nailed? Why indeed? Because if you don't try, then you'll never know. Oh, and because you are worried that other people will laugh at you or think less of you, for having tried and failed. Know that that says more about them than you. It tells you about their feelings of shame around failure. In the future, you'll know to be kind when they encounter a setback, understanding the pain that causes.

May 27

...stop saying I'm sorry for being a strong woman

When Elizabeth started playing rugby in college, she couldn't believe mothers let their daughters play the sport. It was so physical. Every time she made the full-body contact the sport required, she would apologize to the other player. Until her coach explained that she just had to stop saying sorry for playing the game well.

Another thing women don't have to be sorry for on a rugby team? Being unabashedly who they are. Before she played rugby, Elizabeth was self-conscious about her height. She also suffered from an eating disorder. But when she joined the rugby team, she joined a group of women who laughed at their bodies, celebrated their strength, came in all shapes and sizes, and generally breached all the confining norms about what it means to be a woman.

An accumulation of micro-learning moments in rugby added up to the "macro-power person that I am," as Elizabeth says. She's run a big company. But she's had the strength of purpose to step back from that workaholic self to spend more time with her son, coach girls' soccer, found a girl's rugby league in her town, and continue working as a consultant to her old company. No apologies necessary.

We do not need to say "I'm sorry" for being strong!

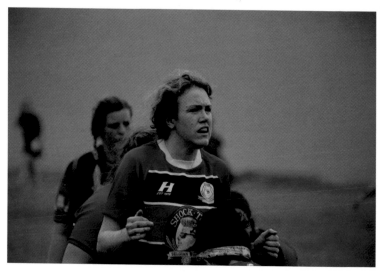

Elizabeth playing rugby. *Credit: Photo courtesy of Elizabeth*

May 28

. . . imposter syndrome

One of the reasons we are often tempted to say "I'm sorry" is that we feel like a fraud. We don't quite feel like we deserve to be at the starting line. You know that sinking feeling that you are not capable enough, despite all evidence to the contrary? A 1978 study by psychologists Pauline R. Clance and Suzanne A. Imes coined the term "imposter syndrome" to describe the internal experience of phoniness that many high-achieving women experience. A feeling aggravated by a society that often treats us like we don't belong in a rugby scrimmage, in corporate leadership, or in a university philosophy department.

Of course, we do belong in all of those places and many of us are more than qualified to be there. The challenge is to step up to the starting line and lay claim to our strength and capacities, both on the field and in the world.

May 29

. . . grow out of your imposter

Here's the thing—feeling like an imposter can stunt our growth. To cultivate a growth mindset requires confidence. You have to be in a state of mind that encourages you to put yourself out there. Maybe we even need to be overconfident at times. It's no secret which of the genders is better at asserting confidence. Our ability to find the learning opportunity inside a failure depends on how secure we feel. When we trust our abilities, we can take the note on what to change and keep moving, without getting mired in self-doubt.

When she was writing a fluffy (in the best way) article about famous people's favorite movies that features their professions, journalist and author Monica Hesse called three times more women than men in her interview process. She ended up quoting many more men than women.

In an answer to the criticism that arose from this gender imbalance, she pointed out that too many of the women she called said they weren't "qualified" to answer; that they weren't expert enough or funny enough about their choices. They literally recommended she talk to someone else, often a man. *Really!?* Accomplished women did not have enough confidence in their . . . movie preferences?

My favorite movie that features running is *Run Lola Run*, a German film from 1998, because the woman runs fast and hard and it's not a stunt, it's just a real, strong woman.

May 30

. . . qualified to be on the green

Golf offers another great window into this "I'm not good enough" phenomenon. In the financial industry (as one example), there's still a lot of business that gets done on the golf course, and as it turns out, men are not always the ones who exclude women's access. Women often exclude themselves.

As Jane, a former pro golfer, says, "Women have no idea how pitiful men's golf games often are . . . Women want to have studied and practiced and be good before they feel comfortable joining." The men don't wait. They'll turn up, even if they've never played before.

Jane turned her talent into a company that helps women penetrate the inner sanctum of the golf green.

May 31
. . . the V-word

I wonder if women shy away from what might be perceived as overconfidence, because they've met one too many men spreading his brash bluff around. We don't want to grow ourselves some balls, as that worn-out saying goes, because we don't want to be like that. Yet we feel like imposters, in a world where braggadocio is too often effective.

We need to grow into our vaginas.

Vagina, as a word, is so underused that when I use it here, it feels a little shocking. Vagina makes me think of the artist Georgia O'Keeffe's fierce, feminine-power flowers. There, I said it again. I actually say vagina out loud more often than you'd think.

The word rhymes with my name. Go ahead. Say it out loud.

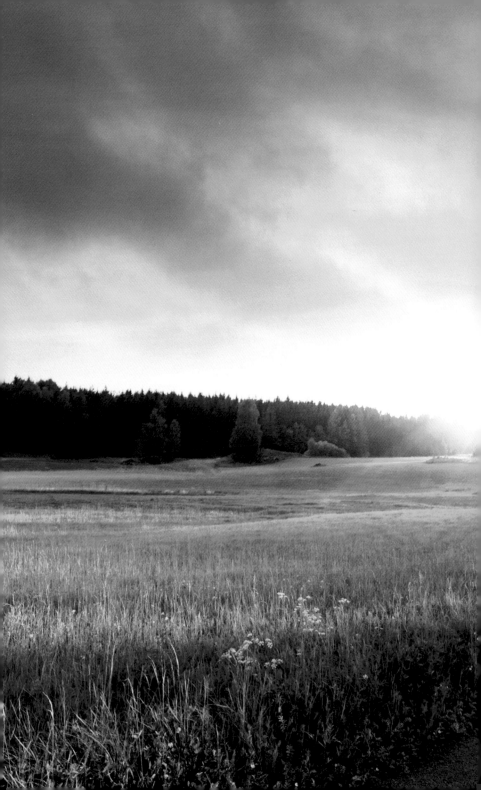

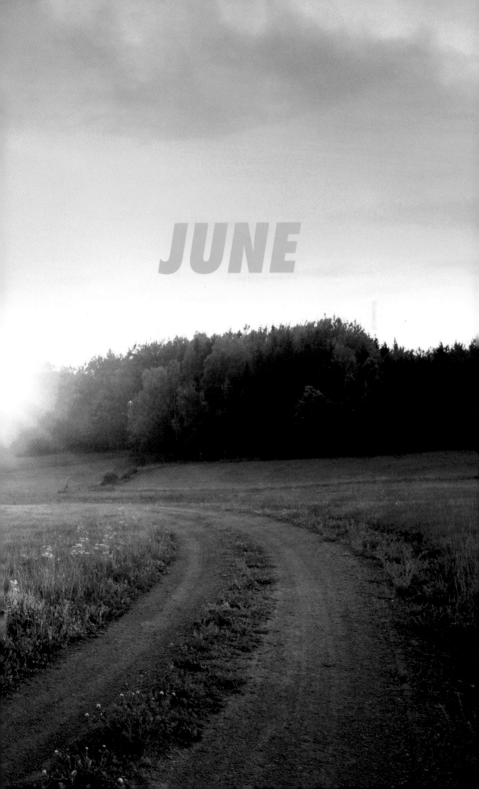

JUNE

June 1

... fearless

I see that word used in so many different contexts now. I wonder what it means. What is fearless beauty? To be fearless is a state of being that marketers now think we should all strive for. Really? Is fearlessness even possible? More—is it desirable?

Setting aside the big, wide world of justifiable fears (poverty, war, cancer, and such), each of us has our own personal drawer cluttered with an assortment of diverse and particular fears. While many of them are related to our physical well-being (or someone else's), for most of us, after living with the food and shelter we need in a relatively conflict-free situation, the majority of the fears that float at the top of our minds are related to the possibility of failure and humiliation.

Despite my poor showing in that recent trail half marathon, I signed up for a 30K on trails that will be at least as challenging, and will be run at altitude. As I write this, it's about five weeks away. I'm scared. Silly, right? What's the worst that can happen? I'll walk. The event will take a really, really long time. I'll be disappointed in myself. Again. Other people (maybe you reading this now) will think I'm a bad runner, or too old for running.

But that won't stop me from running it. I tell myself, "Fall down seven times, and stand up eight."

June 2

. . . bon courage

The French have a saying, *bon courage*. Which they use to mean variously—have courage, keep going, looking strong, you can do it, go get 'em, etc. If you're ever running in Quebec or France, you might hear it. Translated literally it means, *good courage*.

Rather than be fearless, let's have good courage.

June 3

. . . sensible shoes

Here's another of my fears—that I will become *that* woman in sensible shoes. One word—orthopedic.

A couple of years ago, I bought a pair of super-comfortable sandals. Friends and even strangers on the street kept telling me, "Those look comfortable."

My sandals were Thierry Rabotin, which sounds French and rhymes with Louboutin. So how could they be dowdy? Still, I felt a twinge of distress every time I wore them. They hadn't been anointed by the sensible-hip trend, the way Uggs, Fit Flops, and Birkenstocks had been. Was I really going to let that social-marketing fact get inside my head?

I was. I did not have the good courage to wear sandals that made me feel frumpy in others' eyes.

June 4

. . . high heels

Since we're talking about shoes, I'll admit that I have a weakness for the vertiginous kind. High heels often get a bad rap in feminism. You may be thinking, why is she even mentioning high heels in a book for strong, athletic women? That argument goes along these kind of lines: Heels diminish women (oppress and enslave are stronger words some use) by crushing her feet into unnatural and uncomfortable positions, by making it difficult to walk, to keep up with men, or to run away.

True that. . . . And yet, I feel powerful and sexy in them, too, as I stride down the street in my tall, Amazonian guise.

To paraphrase *Psalms*: There's a time for running shoes and a time for high heels.

June 5

. . . let's get red in the face

Whether or not we are willing to wear a pair of ugly shoes seems like an insignificant fear. Yet it signifies the larger issue, that our fears are often related to how others perceive us.

Back in my attorney days, I used to go to the gym in the same building as the law firm. Even though I'd take a shower before heading back up to the office, I was usually still pretty red in the face when I got to my desk. A female colleague once asked me why I allowed myself to get that flushed, as if it was something I ought to correct. It hadn't even occurred to me that I might be judged for my physical exertion.

Her question gave me pause, but ultimately I like how my beating heart paints my face. Even then, before I'd discovered my passion for running, I knew that I wasn't going to stop pushing myself physically just to fit in with some ice-queen attorney standard.

I left that law firm and you know the rest.

June 6

. . . we all fear

The thing about our fears, big, small, rational, irrational—and who decides that anyway?—is that we all have them. Our fears may be different, but we share the experience. We just don't always remember that.

June 7

. . . the hare and the frogs

Here's one of those seventeenth century French fables, on fear:

A hare was pondering in his burrow (because what else is there to do in a burrow, if not ponder?). The hare was mired in a profound ennui. Fear ate at the insides of this sad animal.

He thought to himself: Naturally fearful people are so unfortunate. They don't know how to enjoy the least morsel to their benefit. There is no pure pleasure. They are under attack from all sides. That's how I live. This damned fear keeps me from sleeping. Even if I tried, I'd sleep with eyes open. A wise mind would say, transform your fear. Oh really, fear can be transformed? I think that even humans are scared like me.

So reasoned the hare, while at the same time keeping watch. He was doubtful, worried—a whisper, a shadow, a nothing—all made him feverish.

One day, the melancholy animal, musing in this fashion, heard a slight noise. It was his signal to scuttle back to his den. On his way he passed a swamp. Frogs jumped into the rippled water in an instant. Frogs hurried back to their deep grottos.

The hare said to himself: "Oh! I'm doing to others what's been done to me! My very presence is scaring them. I've set off alarms in the frog's kingdom. Where has this valor come from? How! Animals trembling before me! Have I become a weapon of war?"

The hare continued: "I see now—there's none on earth who is so timid they can't find someone more scared than they are."

June 8

. . . we are all hares and frogs

We are all hiding scared in our burrows on some days and sending someone else hopping into the water on other days.

When our good courage is absent, if we can remember that other people feel the same way, even if they fear different things, then we can stop beating ourselves up for spending the day in our burrow. When our good courage is at our side, make the best of it and share it with others.

In fact, have you noticed that sharing your courage with others often increases your own? I don't mean in that I-triple-dare-you-to-lie-down-on-the-train-tracks way; I mean in that let's-do-this-together-and-we'll-have-more-fun kind of way.

Share some good courage today!

June 9

. . . the world opening on a wave

Trawling the Internet one late night, Hope, an activist labor lawyer and lifetime athlete, booked herself on a surfing trip to Costa Rica. She had never surfed before.

When she got there, she discovered that the majority of the group was a cohort of six women surfers, longtime travel companions, older, married with children, and not her type. Late one night she called the airline from a phone booth to change her ticket. Shutting herself off from experiences and detaching from people was familiar. But the escape route wasn't available. She couldn't change her flight.

Then an unexpected thing happened. The others' courage and energy hooked into Hope. Surfing opened a whole world inside her heart, connecting her to these women who *weren't her type*. Hope says the word she wants to use is *blossomed*, but she hesitates because it sounds kitsch. Apt is how the word sounds to me. And fortunate.

Over the next decade she joined in on the women's annual surfing trips, carving out a place for herself outside of work. While she loves being a lawyer, Hope is clear now that work

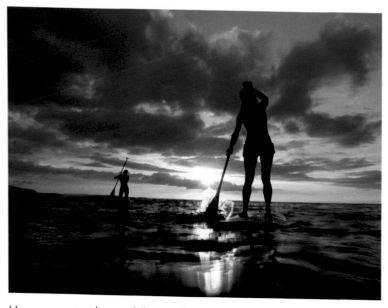

Hope on a standup paddleboard. *Credit: Photo courtesy of Hope*

does not define the whole of who she is. Now she's the type of woman with good courage to share.

June 10

. . . courage to share

You may be thinking: *That Hope, she didn't need those women to be courageous. Look at her. She was booking a trip to learn how to surf for the first time in her mid-thirties, and she was going alone. She already had plenty of courage.*

Our courage is not terribly useful to the rest of the world, if we don't even notice it. How can we share something, if we don't know we have it?

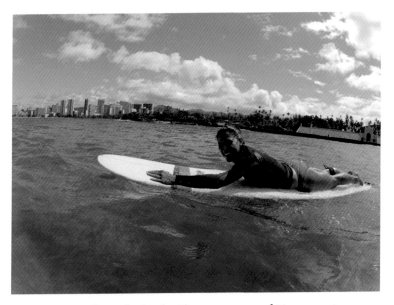

Hope on a surfboard. *Credit: Photo courtesy of Hope*

Hope found what she already had (with a little help from the universe, which left no empty seats on an earlier return flight).

June 11

. . . a true cliché

We all have reservoirs of untapped strength. We have everything we need already inside of us.

Transformation is rarely ever an explosion of the new. Sometimes it takes getting pushed to the edge of our resources, burned out by work and romantic woes, before we tap the source. Other times, it is the slow accumulation of moments of strength, which tips the scales.

Then, one day we understand we are a new person.

June 12

. . . tarps snapping in the wind

One night I was awakened, and then kept awake, by a mystery sound outside; an arrhythmic snapping sound. All night, I wondered what the noise was. In the morning light I saw it was a blue tarp on the roof of an adjacent building.

How could I have failed to recognize that sound? Only a few months earlier I had spent four days fasting alone in the New Mexico desert as part of a vision quest. One of the biggest challenges was the *snap, snap*, snapping of my tarp in the high winds that blew through all day, every day.

I'd brought the tarp to sleep under and shelter myself from the sun, but I neglected to bring the required poles. I left the rudimentary shelter up in case it rained, in which event it seemed like it might offer more protection than the low juniper bushes I was crawling under for their shade.

All day, every day, I'd listened to the *snap, snap*, snapping, as the relentless wind blew and the sun beat down and the desert dust swirled, covering everything, filling my eyes and ears. *Snap, snap*, snapping. *Snap, snap*, snapping. At times I thought I might explode and tear my tarp or myself limb from limb.

I was supposed to be deeply contemplating my life and the universe in the peace of my solitude. Instead, I was allowing an irritant to jangle my nerves and supplant the profound thoughts I thought I ought to be having. Solitude does not equal peace every time, that's for sure.

June 13

. . . solitude refuels

When I realized that the sound that had woken me was a tarp snapping in the wind, I felt a little bit of peace. The next night I missed hearing the sound, because the tarp had been tied down more securely.

I used to hate being alone. It would make me squirrely. Was I relevant, did I still exist if no one saw me? Now I love time by myself. Time when I'm not even reaching out to the world, not emailing, texting, or phoning. I like disconnecting and feeling invisible, a sensation like floating, when it's good. A run alone in the mountains in the early morning when no one is around can be like that. Solitude refuels me, clarifies and heightens my interactions with the world.

June 14

. . . daydreaming

What was I . . .?

We are called to be present in the world. But sometimes, it is a beautiful thing to let our souls take flight. Some days I go out for a run with my mind in the clouds. A trance takes hold when I set out and before I know it I'm back home. I don't quite remember the journey and had no consciousness of effort. But my head is clear and my body is happy.

June 15

. . . boiling brains versus active limbs

Daydreaming doesn't come from boredom. Bored is what we say when we don't want to say how we really feel and why.

Bored is actually antsy. Our minds are moving a mile a

minute and there is no activity to distract us from the thinking we don't want to hear. I'm bored! *No.* I'm thinking too much and it's overwhelming me with—what?—anxiety, self-doubt, a feeling that I am not in the right place, that it is not the right time, or even, that I am not the right person.

We can't outrun our not-boredom, but we can sometimes tame it. Slow the pace of our thoughts. Divert some blood from our boiling brains into our active limbs.

June 16

. . . paying attention on the bike

Biking home from my aerial Pilates class this morning, a woman stepped out in front of me unexpectedly. I swerved widely to avoid her, afterward glancing back over my shoulder to shoot a few stink-eye darts in her direction. By the time I'd returned my eyes to the forward direction, a man was swerving to avoid me. He didn't bother to glare, but I got the message loud and clear about paying better attention.

What a waste of time it is to look backward, even for a moment, at our grievances—not only is it extending our own suffering, but it might cause us to miss out on what's actually happening in front of us.

June 17

. . . catching up with our cat

My partner and I live in Manhattan for nine months of the year, and in California's mountains the other three months. I'm grateful for my good fortune. It feeds both my love of the go-go city and my need to be among trees and rocks and dirt. There are drawbacks, as with anything. One is leaving my friends in New York for extended periods of time.

The other is traveling with our cat and the anxious guilt around the stress we imagine we are putting our cat through. Then there are the almost inevitable scatological events, which usually occur in the taxi on the way to the airport. Then there are flights with turbulence.

Yet we arrive and within moments, our cat has re-adjusted to the new, yet familiar environment. She isn't looking back at her travel grievances.

Meanwhile, we humans take hours, sometimes days, to adjust. And I don't just mean physically—psychologically, too.

This summer, as I'm writing this, we went for our first mountain-bike ride of the season a few hours after we arrived. We adjusted much more quickly; catching up with our cat on our bikes.

June 18

. . . our non-dominant side

During the summer 2012 Olympics, I read about a gold medalist who had improved his hurdling by training ambidextrously. That is, he trained to be able to lead over the hurdles with either leg, something that most champions—even Olympians—cannot do well. Based on the hurdler's story, I decided to improve my mountain biking by learning how to cycle more ambidextrously, which essentially means to be able to click your foot out of your pedal clip with equal ease on both left and right. Instinctively, I have always clipped out with my right foot first. I needed to learn how to do that same thing with my left foot. Developing this ambidextrousness would be enormously helpful in tight situations on the bike. It wouldn't matter if I was falling to the left or right into a prickle bush, because I would be able to escape either pedal with ease.

The project vis-à-vis the mountain bike continues. I've gotten comfortable with left foot leading in no-stress situations, but when the heat is on, it's always my right foot that jumps out of the pedal clip, whether or not it's appropriate to the situation at hand. I'm still ending up in the prickle bushes a fair amount of the time. But I do think my biking is improving. Baby steps.

June 19

. . . my ambidextrous project

I've extended the ambidextrous project to other things, too: unlocking the double bolt to my apartment door; reversing the chain closures on my necklaces; brushing my teeth.

I can't say for sure if there has been any improvement in mental or emotional dexterity, say, or increased creativity. The sheer fact that I was able to reprogram myself, even for a short time, helps me understand the pliable potential of my brain. How much change I'm capable of is up to me.

June 20

. . . blueberry possibility

My grandnan (maternal grandmother) once said to me, "You are like blueberries. So full of possibility."

At the time, I didn't understand. She usually wasn't prone to such Zen-ish statements. So, I have rolled those words around in my brain ever since.

Blueberries are one of the only naturally blue foods (don't be a party-pooper and tell me that they are technically a shade of purple that looks blue). And I love them.

But what's the possibility the berries contain? I still don't know. Yet, I can't help thinking of blueberries anytime I think of possibility, potential, and change.

June 21

. . . the water we swim in

Here's a Zen-ish story: *Two young fish are swimming along. They pass an older fish swimming the other way, who greets them with a nod and says, "Morning, girls, how's the water?" The two young fish say hello, too, and swim on for a bit. Until eventually one of them says, "What's water?"*

We are saturated by media—social and otherwise. Our culture, the way we live, the water we swim in, feels, not just normal, but essential, foundational, and often unchangeable.

But it isn't. Fortunately though, there are always some fish who are aware of the water's quality and speak up. For instance, we have Title IX, a law that requires (among other things) equal access to sports for girls and women in high school and university. Because a lot of people don't seem to notice that sporty girl-fish are getting a lot fewer opportunities at school.

June 22

. . . Title IX waters

Title IX passed in 1972. Yet equal access to sports is still not a reality everywhere.

In the late 1990s, when Becky started playing rugby for the first NCAA Division I women's rugby team, people threw trash at the young women players and sometimes even punched them in the face. Their practice field was unfenced and next to a road, so people regularly walked through their play. Practice often started late, because medieval reenactors were having sword fights on the field. Their rugby coach, a man, told them to be grateful they even had a team. This is after more than twenty-five years of Title IX on the books.

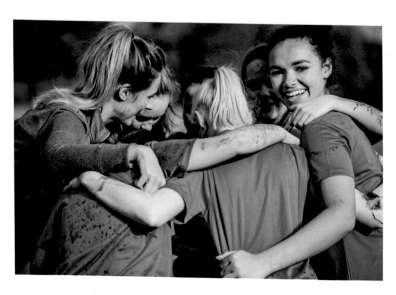

June 23

... rugby pioneer

Becky was always aware of the water in which she swam. As a child, she'd played baseball on the boys' team, because there were no girls' teams on the military base where she grew up. Becky spoke out about how the college's public commitment to her rugby team masked its private disregard. Behind the show of equality, the institution was starving the women's program.

When the local press got wind of Becky's complaints and published a scathing indictment, the athletic department threatened to take away her graduate assistantship, which paid for her education, if she didn't call the newspaper to recant. Becky stood her ground. The school backed down on its threat.

June 24

... once an activist, always an activist

Twenty years have passed since Becky refused to back down. She is still fighting for women and sports, refusing to accept the water we currently swim in. She coaches a women's rugby team, which has won the national championship multiple years in a row. She risks her job on a regular basis to speak

out. She is an advocate through her platform (thefearlesscoach
.org), where she has created a below-the-radar safe-space for
other women coaches who are struggling to share their stories. She doesn't know yet what her network will turn into.
Her first mission is to share little doses of inspiration.

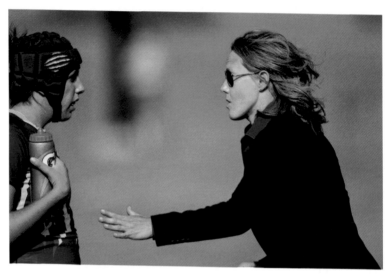

Credit: Photo courtesy of Becky

June 25

. . . Mrs. Tennis Champion

When Serena Williams won Wimbledon (again) in 2018, she
was no longer posted on the board of champions as Miss
S. Williams, but rather Mrs. S. Williams. She got married in
September 2017. Married women are all "Mrs." on the board

of champions at the All England Club. That's some stagnant water we swim in. Even now. And I haven't even gotten into the dust-ups around her attire (fabulous) and her interactions with umpires (unfair).

June 26

. . . well, ride faster

I was communing with my special rock during a trail run, absorbing the heat and letting my thoughts fall into the black swirl behind my eyelids, when I heard a family ride by on mountain bikes. I opened my eyes. The mother was in the lead, and looked uncomfortable on the bike. The father was riding behind his young daughter. She couldn't have been more than eight years old. She rode tentatively.

Father: "Are you even riding?"

(Dear reader, his daughter was obviously riding.)

Daughter: "I am riding."

Father: "Well, ride faster.

How motivating. Maybe that kind of un-encouragement works with some people. But I had the urge to put a stick in the father's spokes.

June 27

. . . biking to college

I learned about Rajni Devi on malala.org. Rajni lives in a small town in India. When she was fourteen, she was supposed to leave school and get married. She fought the cultural norm, bringing home grades so good that she convinced her father to call off the marriage. Now she bikes thirty kilometers (eighteen miles) each way to college. Fortunately, she loves cycling, the same way she loves learning. She has a strong foundation to build on.

June 28

. . . was that tree root always that big?

I took a break from writing these pages to go for a mountain-bike ride, my second of the season. I was feeling a bit frustrated with my writing, or rather, with staring at my computer screen with nothing to write. I was feeling overwhelmed, too, by a world filled with so many fights for women's rights.

Clear blue sky. Bright sun. Light wind. Cool, fresh air. The day couldn't have been more perfect. Even so, for me, the first days out every season are always a lesson in patience. Didn't I ride over these loose rocks with no problem last year? Was that tree root always such a big ledge to get up and over? I know I did it without a thought last summer. I will make it up this hill. *I will make it up this hill.* Breathe hard. Try not to drool from the exertion. I made it up the hill.

I used to get much more frustrated by the two-steps-forward-one-step-back-ness of getting back on my mountain bike each season. Over the years, though, my attitude has adjusted. I focus more on the increments of technical skill that stay with me over the winter, instead of the obstacles I need to relearn. Last year I didn't make that downhill hairpin the first time out. Today, I did. I feel more confident that the skills I've lost will come back. I look beyond where I finished the season the year before and find the new skills I want to aim for in the season to come.

June 29

. . . grateful riding

Refocusing on where I'd done well on my mountain-bike ride was only part of the story when I took that break from writing. The other piece was gratitude. I was out riding for a workout, yes, but exercise can be gotten in many ways that don't involve fresh mountain air. I wasn't required to ride eighteen miles each way to school just to get an education. I was riding for the sheer pleasure of it. What great fortune I was enjoying.

I sat back down to write with new energy and patience.

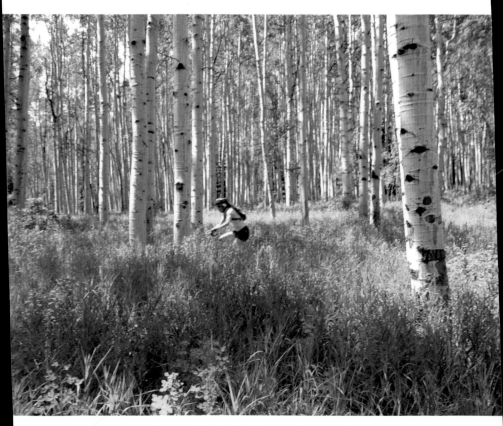

Mountain biking in Vail. *Credit: Noah Samuels*

June 30

... riding over cicadas on your bicycle

In 2013, the United States had a cicada summer. This is the once-in-seventeen-years summer when great swarms of cicadas descend, like biblical locusts. While I'd seen pictures in the newspaper and heard about them, I hadn't seen them until I went for a ride out of Manhattan across the George Washington Bridge and on up to Nyack. As soon as I crossed the bridge into New Jersey, I started seeing the cicadas. Everywhere.

The road was littered with their carcasses, mostly all dead, but a few were crawling slowly across the road. Their bodies were striped, like a wasp's, their wings a translucent brown. The only spots of color that I could see were two red dots above what I took to be their eyes. In places, the air was filled with flying cicadas, more substantial than a large dragonfly and smaller than a hummingbird.

But it was the sound that struck me most. A whining hum, like the sound of fast car tires on the highway, only pitched a half-tone higher. As I rode, the sound swelled and receded like an accordion; moving into my body, filling my senses. Once I'd heard and identified the sound, I could not un-hear it. I could not escape it; at least not until I rode back over the bridge toward home. The cicadas didn't come to the city. The peace and quiet of home felt sweeter than usual.

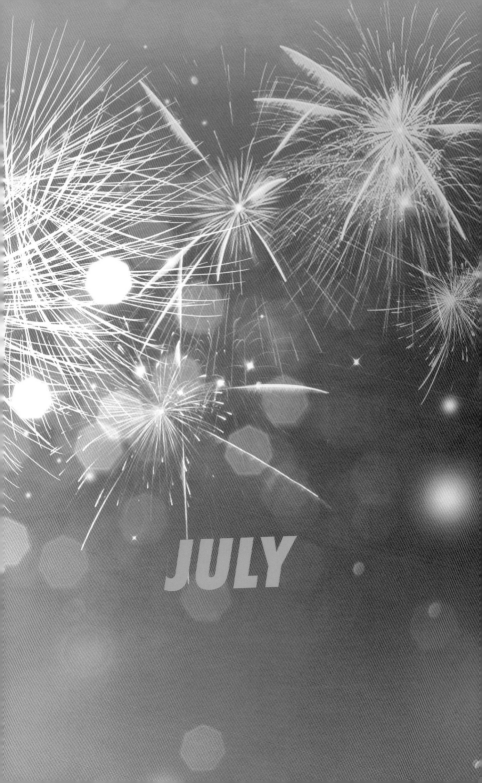

JULY

July 1

... citizenship

The Welsh writer Gwyn Thomas uses the word *citizen* where other writers might use the word *person*. It's a choice I love, for implying, as it does, all the rights and responsibilities of being a person living in community with others.

Citizenship involves belonging, and it's always nice to feel that you are a part of something greater than yourself. We aren't only citizens of countries (or maybe two, as in my case, both of which celebrate country-hood in the month of July), but we are citizens of the communities we are joined to—our workplace, the teams and groups we are part of, our neighborhood, and ultimately, the world.

Let's be good citizens. Look up from this book right now. Smile at the first person whose eye you catch; if you're alone, smile at you.

July 2

... messages from the universe

One night my partner and I were playing Honeymoon Bridge, a card game I won't explain, except to say that there is a trump suit. Usually we choose the trump with a random split of the deck, but this time we decided that since it was random and didn't give an advantage to either player, that the dealer would just decide which suit they *liked* for trump. I chose diamonds. Dealt the hand. Got almost no diamonds. Lost the hand. The next hand, my partner chose clubs. He got a hand full of clubs and I got a hand full of . . . yes . . . that's right . . . diamonds, a game late, of no use whatsoever.

My partner tried to convince me that it was a sign of good things coming to those who wait. Sure. But he didn't have to wait. He got his clubs right when he needed them. Besides, if the good things come when they are no longer useful or wanted, what's the point? I began angst-ing that this was exactly how my life always was and so on.

Then, he said patiently, it's not a sign of anything. We played a couple more hands and each of us won as much as we lost.

It's easy to confound the inside of our mind with a message from the universe. This run isn't going well; therefore, the universe is telling me that I'm a useless person. This run is going well; therefore, the universe is applauding. Not everything is a sign. Sometimes the world is just random.

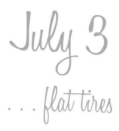

July 3

... flat tires

Then again, sometimes the universe does send a message.

There have been whole years I've gone without a flat tire. And then . . . it's early in the morning. I'm tired, feeling overstretched physically and emotionally. Not only is it the one year anniversary of the death of my beloved cat, whose invisible presence still shows up on my pillow at night sometimes; it's the day I'm leaving for Toronto, to be part of their Fringe Festival 2013, to perform a piece I've written. It's the first time my new venture into playwriting and performing is going really public (as in, not just for friends and family). I'm trying to decide whether to cut my bike ride in the park short. Usually I ride three loops of Central Park, but I'm seriously considering cutting back to two loops. I'm not good at taking it easy, at cutting a workout short. Nor am I good at easing into things, starting slowly. Rather, I'm an expert at self-wear-and-tear, at going until possibly I've been going too long. As I came round to the end of my second loop, I thought, *Oh what the hell, do the third.*

Then, I got a flat tire.

July 4

. . . crying in public

During that extended stay in Toronto, while I took part in the Fringe Festival, I rented a kick-around-the-city bike. Most of the time, the bike was a boon and I loved the feeling of wheeling around. But a couple of times it rained. Not just a drizzle, but torrentially, as in, this-is-the-worst-since-1954-subways-shut-down-and-power-outages rainstorm. That storm happened on the day I got a bad review of my play, which called it banal. So there was a real storm to match my internal storm. It didn't matter that another highly respected theatre reviewer had glowed about my show the day before. I was devastated. And I was stuck at a theatre, the rain sheeting down.

After being stormed out of dinner with a friend and going to another play, in hopes that the worst of the storm would pass, I decided there was nothing for it but to bike home in the deluge. My thank-heavens-it-was-black dress was soaked through in a matter of moments and gained four inches in water-weight length. I was cold. I was overwhelmed by my first experience participating in a Fringe Festival. I was lonely and hungry. And I was feeling stupendous-level defeat. I started crying on the bike.

The rain fell so hard that I couldn't feel my tears. Engulfed by my misery and awheel in the storm, I found the space I needed inside the movement of cycling to let my internal typhoon wash through me.

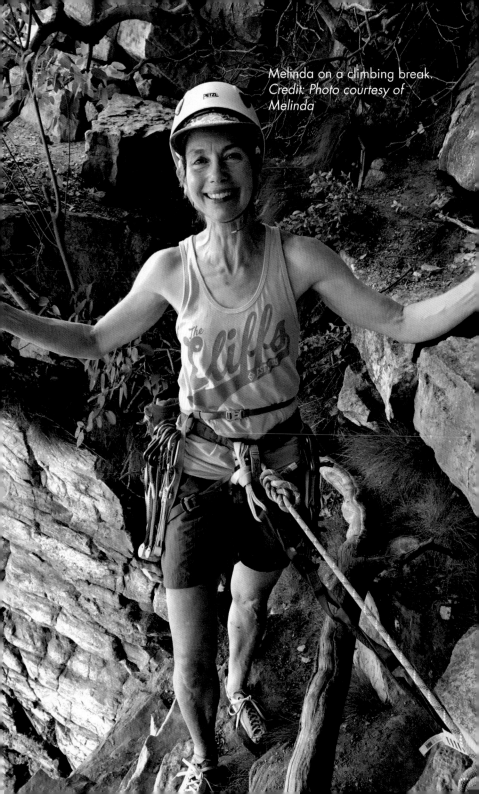

Melinda on a climbing break.
Credit: Photo courtesy of Melinda

July 5

. . . a sentence in a textbook

Melinda was raised on a farm in Texas. She was riding horses at four. At seventeen, she herniated two disks and tore her hamstring in ballet. Prompted by that injury, when she hit university she wanted to study how the body worked. She started working part-time at a physiology and biochemistry lab in Houston. She loved the work, but realized it was too indoors for her. "I could see years and years of my life fade away for a sentence in a textbook."

Melinda changed course for medical school and found her way to anesthesiology. Because, "Who wouldn't want to know how to intubate?" She worked at prominent hospitals. Eventually she noticed that a lot of her patients weren't getting better on the panoply of prescribed medications, which led her to discover acupuncture. After years of incorporating traditional pain management and acupuncture at private ambulatory facilities, she's practicing acupuncture full-time now. Never one to slow down, she's also studying for her diploma in mountain medicine, which is just one of the many outdoor medical and rescue certifications she's pursued.

Melinda's love of the outdoors has guided and fed her throughout her life. She learned to ski when she was twenty-eight. She's a self-taught telemark skier and every winter she takes new PSIA (Professional Ski Instructors Association) courses. In her sixties, she's set her sights on another new thing, ski mountaineering races.

July 6

. . . to see who we are

Melinda needs an active life. "No matter our age, we need to be strengthening our bodies," she says. "Why wouldn't we be trying to stay strong?"

She wants to test her outer limits, to see how it feels in her own body. In the same way, she likes hard patient-cases with complicated issues for her to solve. Melinda's passion for the outdoors and her intense curiosity about how the human body works nourish each other. "That's why we do this stuff. Because we have to dig deep and see who we are."

July 7

. . . mountain biking in French

Fear is probably the biggest thing that stands in the way of achieving our goals. One of the things that interfere with my progress in speaking French is my fear that I'll say the wrong word or muff the pronunciation. So, I silence myself, instead of trying. At a certain point, I realized that I was holding my own self back for fear of looking dumb. Nothing more. And really what was I scared of? Do I think of non-English speakers who add flourishes to my native language as stupid? No. I made the decision to forge ahead with a bolder attitude. The approach is more fun and it's helped my French.

Balking at a tight corner this morning on my mountain bike, I saw with renewed clarity how similar the fear was. The worst danger I faced on this particular turn was that I'd ride off into the bushes. I wasn't fearful of hurting myself (though often I am). I was just scared of looking foolish. Even though I was by myself.

Recognizing the difference between our healthy fears, which keep us safe, and our other fears, which keep us in a cage, is not the work of one day. We have to actively reassess what makes us fearful and why.

July 8

. . . nothing fearless about it

When the athletic department at Becky's university discovered the hockey coach's psychological abuse, it convened a meeting with all the rest of the coaches. The department fired the hockey coach, but also told the rest of the coaches to say that they knew nothing. That was not okay with Becky, the rugby coach. When she said so, the Associate Athletic Director told her to shut her mouth.

"I felt my face getting red. My heart was beating like crazy. My mouth was dry. I started crying. There was nothing fearless about my reaction," Becky says.

Despite her fear—she documented everything that happened. She contacted the Title IX coordinator at the college and made sure the vice president knew, even though it became apparent they would do nothing. Becky felt sick going to work, but she continued to be a thorn in their side. She was accused of forcing a pro-women agenda on her players (who are women). She faced a tribunal for her supposed subversive and divisive behavior, but with one of the top employment lawyers in the country fighting for her, she's kept her job . . . so far. She feels vulnerable and hunted. She persists.

July 9

. . . take fear's hand

When we say fearless, we don't really mean without fear. Fearless is the word we use when we persist, even while we're crying and red in the face and full of fear, but we know that to be our fullest, most powerful selves, to live our most meaningful and engaged life, we have to take fear's hand and walk with it. Our fear is less than our resolve.

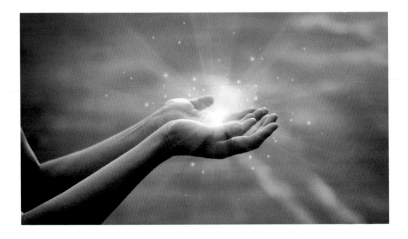

July 10

. . . sunburn

I am fair-skinned and have had my share of sunburns in my life. I have laid in bed chilled and fevered from the sun's hot gaze. As a teenager, I thought the best base for a nice suntan was a burn.

The worst sunburn I remember was at summer camp. I went to an all-girls camp, which I loved. The sunburn happened on the last day of a canoeing trip. I had French-braided my hair and forgotten to cover my ears. They were swollen and aflame. I was awake half the night with the pain.

When I finally feel asleep, I dreamed that my fellow campers and even the counselors were using my ears to heat water. At first it was just small cups of water, for tea or to wash their faces. I would dip my flaming ear in their mug and the water would boil.

I still wonder if the dream had any deeper meaning, or if all dreams have meaning or only some.

The other day I was out on a long trail run and realized I'd forgotten to put sunscreen on my ears. I enjoyed a quick scroll through my summer-camp memories, while I took a sunscreen application break.

July 11

. . . wear sunscreen

Do you remember that Kurt Vonnegut Internet hoax? The one where a commencement speech titled "Wear Sunscreen" was attributed to him. Vonnegut didn't write the speech, it turned out, which we all should have known; cute-but-wise is not his style. That was the first time I remember being taken in by a widespread Internet hoax.

The advice wasn't wrong. Sunscreen is important. It keeps our skin young and prevents cancer, so we can keep on playing outside. But we do need to check our facts.

July 12

. . . does the eagle shed its beak?

Some years after the Vonnegut Hoax, a yoga teacher told my class that she had just learned that when eagles get to be about forty years old, that they either have to go through the painful process of knocking their own beaks off, so the beak can grow back strong and healthy, or they will die. Apparently by that point their forty-year-old beaks are no longer strong enough to capture prey, and they starve to death. She told us the story as a nature-showing-the-way kind of cautionary tale, because she herself had just turned forty. I was early in my forties.

The story sounded intriguing, not just for its metaphorical value, but also as one of those amazing-but-true things that happen in the animal kingdom. So, I looked it up.

Internet hoax.

Too bad. Because the message of the story is true: We can't let ourselves get stale and averse to change as we age. Sometimes we need to knock off our beaks and start again.

July 13
. . .the thrill of flip-flops

I couldn't wear flip-flops until I was about forty. I never wore them as a child and by the time I was twelve I couldn't. That web of skin between my big toe and second toe was simply too delicate to wear them without pain. Once, in my early twenties, on a trip in Africa to mark the end of law school, I had to buy a pair of emergency flip-flops. Walking the short distance between the cabin where my friend and I were staying and the showers, I started bleeding between my toes.

How I envied those who could wear flip-flops. They are insouciant, much sexier than straight-across straps.

Miraculously, somewhere around the age of forty, I was suddenly able to wear flip-flops (better than knocking a beak off).

There's nothing like finishing a triathlon, or a long trail run, and slipping a strap between my toes on the way to sweet-potato fries and ice cream. It's the cherry-thrill on top of the tough workout.

July 14

. . . does happiness require suffering?

When asked in an interview if he was happy in the ring, Georges St-Pierre, a former world champion ultimate fighter, answered that in the moment of the fight he was not happy. He was too filled with all the various fears he faced in a match. But afterward, when the match was over: yes, he was happy. St-Pierre then referred to the idea (most often credited to Buddhism) that happiness is really just the moments when we experience the relief from suffering.

When I first heard that I thought, *How dismal*. And yet, at the same moment, I experienced a visceral sensation of the truth of what he was saying. Now, I'm no ultimate fighter, nor am I a world champion of anything, but on the miniature stage of my own life, it certainly feels like a good portion of what makes me happy also makes me suffer; and that the happy part isn't actually possible without the suffering. And you know I'm not just talking about our sports.

July 15

. . . joyful suffering

I have vivid, full-body memories of the starting lines of events I've competed in. I'm scared to the verge of tears. I'm wondering if I can even finish this challenge I've brought upon myself. Then I run (or swim and bike and run, or ski) for what feels like forever, suffering a good deal of the way. But, when I am finished, I feel flooded with elation. A kind of elation I only feel when the accomplishment has involved effort at the level of pain.

July 16

. . . failure feels better if I've suffered

Even failure is easier to bear if I've suffered. After a few years of trying, I thought I'd conquered once and for all the little portion of a mountain-bike climb that was my nemesis (you'll notice I have any number of mountain-biking nemesis rocks and steeps). This particular year, I tried it several times and just couldn't make it all the way. Maybe the rocks got rearranged, or that sand was looser, spinny-er (yes, I made that word up). Maybe I wasn't as strong as before. I was frustrated with myself and kept thinking I wasn't trying hard enough. My last day out, I gave it one more try. And this time, not only did I not make it up; I crashed sideways on my bike trying. Not only had I *failed*, but I was also bruised and scraped. The thing is, I felt better about the failure. Why?

I had given it my best shot.

July 17

. . . running away from suffering can feel worse

As Kelly, an aerial arts instructor, once told me, "I know what it feels like to run away from my fear and I know what it feels like to meet it head-on. The suffering is worse in the running away."

We're not talking just about sports, of course, but everything in life that's hard to come by, which are often also the very things that bring us the most happiness. Think love and relationships (as I'm sure you have), or how about passion and career?

The math is slippery though. The relationship between suffering and happiness is not always proportional. More suffering doesn't equal more happiness. Not all the time. How do we know what the optimal amount of suffering is to achieve our highest happiness?

I don't know the answer for you. For me, it's an ongoing experiment on myself. Fine tuning the dial. Sometimes I get it wrong and I've just plain suffered and am unhappy. But other times . . . make room for my joy.

July 18

. . . learning to trust

I had my old mountain bike for seventeen years. More than a piece of equipment, she was my first faithful trail-riding companion. For most of those years, we didn't spend a lot of time together. I loved her, but didn't trust her (or myself!). Then, in the last few years before we parted, I discovered what trust could look like between us. I let her ride through things I thought were impossible. Rocks. Roots. Ditches. Downhills. Single tracks.

One year it was a bridge repair down in the Euer Valley, one of my standard favorites. The old bridge washed out in the spring. The cobbled-together repair was a narrowing bridge with two step-ups, where one fat plank rested on top of another. On my first attempt, I walked my old bike across. My second pass I let her ride the obstacle. And when *we* made it over, my adrenaline surged and I felt such a full body flush of relief I almost fell off my bike.

Every year she gently showed me the places where it wasn't the terrain getting in my way, but my mind. My bike reminded me that my own fear is often my biggest obstacle. This is a message that never gets old and continues to resonate long after a ride is over. I need to *WOOP* that.

July 19

. . . I am worthy

I loved my old mountain bike. How could I ever leave her for another? Well, it turned out that while we'd been enjoying each other's company, bike technology had rocketed skyward. New terrain-adjustable hydraulic suspension systems. Disc brakes. Wider handle bars. Groovy seats that move out of the way for downhills. Taller wheels.

I don't need fancy tech, I thought.

I rode a little on a bike my partner was test-riding. *Oh. That was different* . . . Better. Still, I thought, I don't need a better bike. By which I really meant—I'm not worth better.

I'm not? Yes I am!

July 20

. . . grit and grace

As much as I loved my old bike, she had one more lesson to teach me. She'd already taught me how trusting her (and myself) overcame obstacles (and my fear). That was the grit part.

But I still needed to learn the grace bit, which is the moment of accepting our skills and talents and gifts; of respecting our capabilities. I rode well enough that a new bike was going to make a difference. Why maintain unnecessary obstacles? In my case it's because some piece of my brain wants to smack me down anytime I think I might be good at something. Pride comes before the fall and all that old business. My mind is comfortable when it's trash talking me.

Grace is the part where we say to ourselves, with humility and curiosity: I'm great. There's space for everyone's greatness. Mine certainly isn't better. Excellence is dynamic. We need to be open to the next challenge.

Grit and grace. Failure and flight.

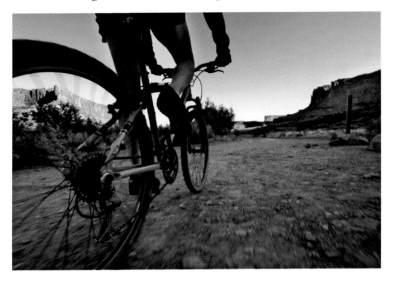

July 21

. . . pre-race evacuation

Some grit: When I'm nervous about an athletic event coming up in a few hours, my body generally sends me to the bathroom quite a few times. My pre-challenge anxiety is made manifest via my bowels. I know that's actually the effects of the stress-induced norepinephrine, but I think it's my body's way of preparing me for what I'm about to do. So it won't distract me while I'm in the midst of a long trail run.

Much of the time our bodies know just what we need.

July 22

. . . talking about intimate body functions

As athletes (really, as people), we need to get comfortable talking about how our body is functioning (even if our talking starts out as an Internet search). After all, our bodies are talking to us and it's worth listening if we want to stay active.

July 23

. . . shame

There's already more than enough shame to go around. Our bodies in all their strength and fragility, beauty and messiness do not deserve to be shamed.

Ever.

July 24

. . . sewage backed up in the basement

That's what body shame is like. Except it's easier to get rid of the effluvia in our basement than it is in our mind.

July 25

. . . body talk

Have you had this experience?

It's a beautiful summer day. Let's say it's an outdoor yoga and music festival. You're hanging out with girlfriends, doing vinyasa, working on your alignment. How wonderful.

Except for this: "My legs are too big for skinny jeans." And, "I like these yoga pants because my butt doesn't look big." And, "I resent my mother for not passing on her breasts to me. Mine are so small." And, "My stomach's not flat enough." Plus the angst over what to eat and the riveting discussion of how many calories are in our typical lunch.

How much of our lives have been spent in these sorts of trite discussions? What a waste. Truly. Let's not fritter away our precious time.

July 26

. . . speaking of intimate things

I don't have a name for my vagina, do you? (Yes, I had to bring the word back.) I hadn't thought to name mine until a friend told me that her grandmother calls hers Mitsy. Makes me want to call mine Regina, which also rhymes with Mina (if you're thinking of the city in Saskatchewan). Is that coincidence, or confirmation of the royal power between my legs? What name would you give (or have you already given) your vagina?

July 27

. . . the quicksands of feminism

Is naming our vaginas feminist?

Most athletic women consider themselves feminist. But the ways in which their feminine power is expressed, other than the physical strength of their athleticism, are myriad. We each have our own "I-know-it-when-I-see-it" definition of feminism and our definition is not always in harmony with another's. Trying to nail down a definition, we find ourselves running uphill in quicksand.

What's important is this: celebrating and supporting our sisters' power; and regularly reexamining how we manifest our own feminism in the world, so our lives are an expression of our best, most up-to-date version. Just as we looked to our mothers, there are generations to come who will look to us for their own roadmap, whether we know they're watching or not.

July 28

. . . terrifying our mothers

"Everything I did terrified my mother," says Tamara, an ordained interfaith minister and healer. "She was fearful of life in general, water in particular. But the more I did, the more adventurous I became."

When Tamara learned how to swim, she felt like she was overcoming not only her own fears, but also her mother's. She didn't get into water sports until she was an adult. The first time she went flying down the face of a wave on a surfboard, she was hooked.

July 29

. . . letting our children terrify us

Like her mother before her, Tamara is daunted by some of the things her children do. Unlike her mother, she passed a sense of adventure onto her children. She encouraged them to terrify her on a regular basis. Her youngest was practicing rollovers in a kayak in Belize at eight years old. In addition to Belize, she took them to Peru, the Galapagos, Mexico, India, Thailand, South Africa, and Zimbabwe.

They're grown now, but they carry their mother's courage and boldness with them.

July 30

. . . the cycle of empowerment

The more we do or try, the more empowered we become. Tamara's surfing pushed her out into the world in a new way. She started to take surf vacations on her own. Emboldened, this led to more and more solo travel. Her open, adventurous nature didn't stop at sports and travel.

She brought that same spirit to her work. She started her career as an occupational therapist. A further massage certification introduced her to non-Western energy healing protocols—polarity therapy, Reiki, mysofascial therapy, unwinding. In Peru, she encountered shamanic traditions and trained with the Andean priests. Each new field of knowledge she explored led her to another.

Now, as an ordained interfaith minister from the Center for Sacred Studies practicing in Massachusetts, some of the most rewarding work she does is sitting in council circles with girls. Passing the cycle of empowerment onto the next generation.

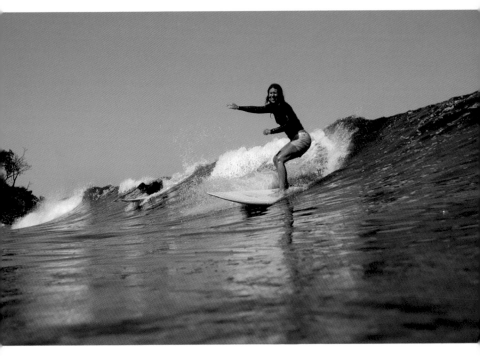

Tamara surfing. *Credit: Cat Slatsinsky*

July 31

. . . meaning and frivolity

For sure, feminism is about cycles of empowerment. But there has to be some fun about it, too. To be mindful in our lives does not mean we are always serious. In fact, we can be mindfully frivolous.

Meaningful frivolity. Frivolous meaning. Serious meaninglessness.

Our feminism can be ferocious and light, just like the best runs.

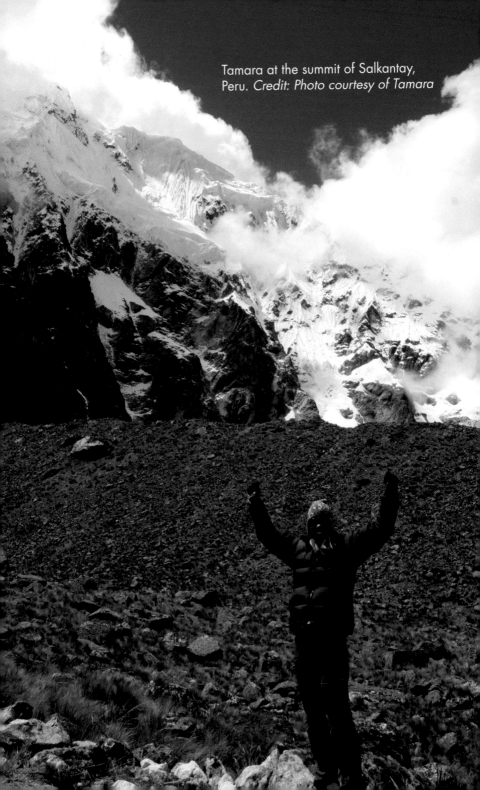

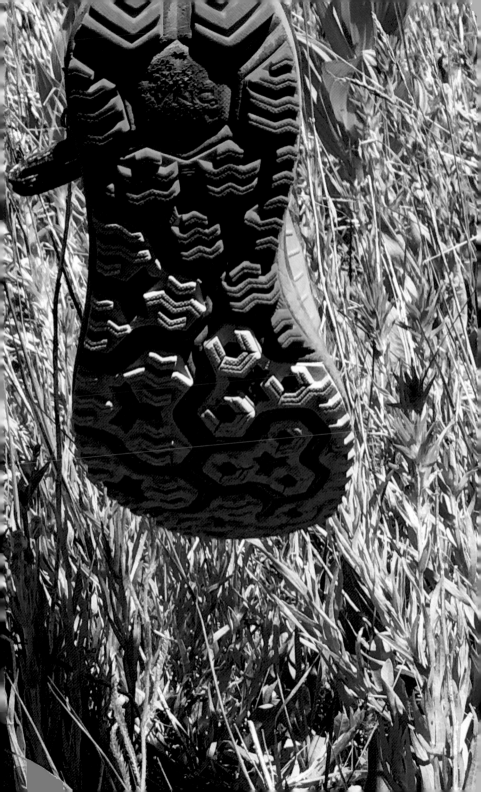

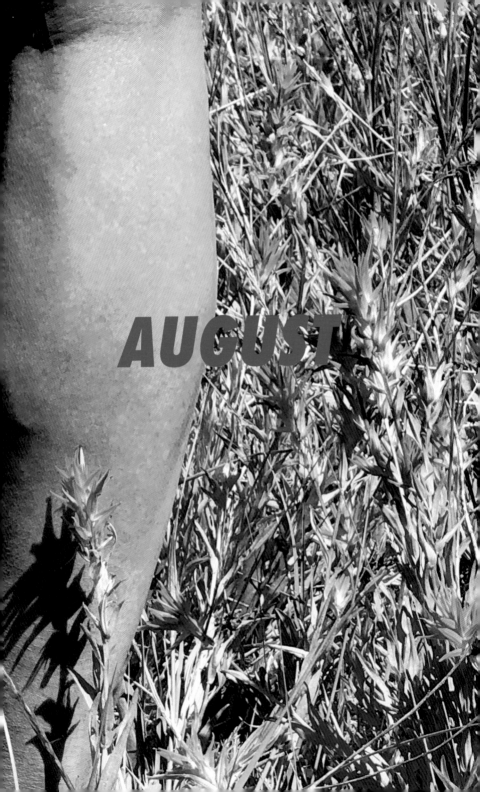

AUGUST

August 1

. . . rocks

During a period when my running mileage was reduced because of the neuromas in my foot, I turned to mountain biking as a substitute for my trail running.

Before I got comfortable on the mountain bike (and even now sometimes), I used to wake up anxious about the ride I was about to do. Some days I have my riding mojo. And the very next day I have one foot on the ground and my heart is jumping around in my chest. Where I ride in California, the major obstacles are rocks (okay—steepness too, as I've mentioned).

On the days I have it, I talk to my bike. If I didn't need to keep both hands on the handlebars, I'd probably pat the crossbar, like the flanks of a horse. Good girl. You go girl. I know you've got this, Will. That's her name. It's the diminutive of Willamina, the great-great aunt for whom I was named Mina.

August 2

. . . diminutives

I've always felt the tiniest bit ripped off that I didn't get the full name Willamina. Instead my parents gave me two diminutive names: Mina Beth. What a world of possibility I would have had, if I'd been named Willamina Elizabeth. I could have been Will, Willie, Willa, Eliza, Lizzie, Liza, Liz, Bette, Bess.

Would my life have been any different?

August 3

. . . nicknames

When I was a child my parents called me Boo, short for The Boozer, which was apparently the name given to me by the neighborhood children when I was just learning how to walk. Apparently, I cruised around at parties, hanging onto chair and sofa cushions, pausing at the cocktail and side tables that were just my height to take sips of drinks.

I grew to hate the nickname, which felt babyish, and put a stop to its use during my surly teen years.

Yet now, I wish for someone to call me Boo.

Nicknames feel different from diminutives. They come bearing history and often love, whereas diminutives are simply shorthand.

So, if we run into each other on the trails, feel free to call me Boo.

August 4

. . . hurtling into the next fall

When I was a child, my mother liked to say that I was never without a bandage or scab on my knee. I was one of those kids constantly hurtling into the next fall.

Some days when I have a run-in with a branch or rock on my bike, I feel like a tough, insouciant badass; that I am grabbing life by the horns. No way am I slowing down.

But other days, when I'm left with scrapes and bruises blooming on my legs or arms, the hurt hooks into a cascade of deeper emotions nesting against my heart. Why can't I even do the simplest thing without getting into a scrape? Why am I clumsy? Unfeminine? I feel an overwhelming sense of futility. As if my hurtling around has nothing to do with making the most out of life. I'm no more than a dog chasing its tail, or worse, a chicken with its head cut off.

Both are true and neither is true.

August 5

. . . waiting for life to start

In Louise Glück's poem "August," two girls sit in their backyard on a late summer day dreaming of a life to come, certain that what they are living isn't yet exactly right, isn't the real thing. "Our lives were stored in our heads./ They hadn't begun."

We all know the feeling of waiting for life to start, of living inside our heads, as if life itself is still pending. But life isn't waiting for us, it's happening now, for real.

To paraphrase Samuel Beckett's play *Waiting for Godot*, we are born astride the grave, the light gleams an instant.

Be present for the light.

August 6

. . . the symphony is still playing

Back on January 5, we talked about waiting to feel 100 percent; the idea that our bodies are like a symphony tuning up, but never playing the piece. Now again, in this slowed-down month of summer, we have the space to cycle back to that reflection from another perspective. We live on the frictionless boundary between what is real, what is intended, and what is hoped for. This boundary is our engagement with life; the musical accompaniment on our road.

August 7

. . . choosing between the stick and the gift

I went for a trail run with my partner and three thirty-somethings I'd never run with before. Squaw Valley to Sugarbowl. Fourteen miles. Close to four thousand feet of elevation gain. Just shy of four hours of running. I had trouble with the initial three-mile climb and then lost my focus. All I could see was that I wasn't good enough. I was old. Weak. Out of shape. I probably weighed too much. Plus, my partner, who is monstrously strong, but comes by his strength with a lower volume of training than I put in, was way ahead of me.

I was in the middle of gorgeous landscape that ought to have taken my breath away. I was with a friendly group of people, filled with good cheer, who could care less that I was slower. But I couldn't notice any of it. I was filled with disappointment in myself.

A few hours after I finished the run, I had collected my mental and emotional state enough to see what a colossal waste of energy all that beating up on myself had been. I missed the opportunity in the moment. I had made my run into a beating stick, instead of a gift and pleasure.

August 8

... more compare, more despair

Remember that 30K I signed up for after the disappointing trail half-marathon? Well, the 30K happened. But before I tell you about it, there's the part where I'm still trying to figure out my bad habit of comparing myself to my partner. Because we were both signed up for the 30K.

In the essay "Love Your Frenemy," in *Aeon*, Sara Pratasi writes that love and envy are flip sides of the same coin. We are most likely to compare ourselves to those closest to us. This resonated with me. I know I'm not alone in the struggle, and if we've partnered with someone fabulous and talented (which is a pretty great view to have of one's life companion), then the bar will always feel high. We are in a double bind when we compare ourselves to our partners. We love them for their winning personalities and talents. We can also envy those same qualities.

Here's a snippet of my inner dialogue when I'm in despairing comparison mode—say, because my partner has passed me in a race: *Life is too unfair. Why do men have it so much easier in the world? Why do I try at all? What's the point of even training? I'll never be good enough.*

That is not the inner monologue of someone who is putting in a best effort.

August 9

. . . always root for, not against

My partner has pointed out that the way I compete with him means I'm rooting against him. I want him to be slower than me, so that I can feel good. I've tried nuancing. I want us both to do the best we can. And I want my best to be better. This line of logical reasoning is not a credit to me. Being competitive is not a bad thing. But it's only healthy, when, as tennis great Chris Evert counsels, we can respond with the same aplomb whether we win or lose.

That's my mission. It's not impossible. I accept.

August 10

. . . letting go at 10K

Which brings me to the 30K in 2018. It featured technical mountain trails at altitude, with lots of climbing. For the week before the run, I was in mental prep mode, counseling myself to just let it go. Let go of my competitive desire to do better. Let go of my tendency toward self-sabotage. Reclaim my power.

Easier said than done.

Race day. The smoke from California forest fires is the worst it's ever been (some volunteers at aid stations are

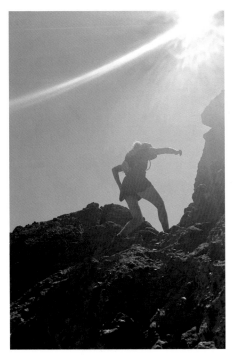

At the top of Castle Peak with a sunburst.
Credit: David Foster

wearing face masks). My partner gives me a hug and kiss before we start. I press play and start listening to Krista Tippett podcasts, something I've never done during an event. Off I go, ahead. After a few miles, my partner passes me. Off he goes, leaving me in the dust. I will not fall apart. I will not fall apart. I'm listening to a podcast about love in politics. At around 10K, I see my partner far ahead of me up a hill. I am overwhelmed by the small-heartedness of my competitive streak. How can I not just be proud of his strength? I want to catch up to him, and say, "Have a great race. You're amazing!" But he's too far away. I feel lighter. Like maybe I've let go. But, like pretty much every moment in life, there's a lot of running left to do.

August 11

. . . running 20K more

At the first aid station, I run through. He's stopped for water. A couple of miles later, on the steepest downhill switchbacks, he waves to me from one switchback above me. He's cheerful. I'm already pretty spent. I'm sure he's going to catch and pass me soon. I use his imminence as incentive to keep going. Not because I want to beat him anymore. I've accepted that's not possible and it's fine. I just want to do my own best time.

Two more grueling hours pass on the trails. He doesn't pass me. Mostly I'm alone. I listen to inspiring interviews with incredible people; with Cory Booker, a US Senator I've long admired; with Robin Wall Kimmerer, a botanist whose specialty is moss; with Luis Alberto Urrea, a writer and poet; and with the great cellist, Yo-Yo Ma.

I finish in 3:53. I'm second in my age group (same as at the half marathon, when I wasn't happy) and tenth among women.

August 12

. . . compete and let go

How do I feel now? Relieved. Surprised. Pleased. Competitive. Displeased with my competitiveness. Uncertain about whether I actually let go. Not sure I fully embodied Chris Evert's advice.

When it comes to my partner, finding the balance between my competitive spirit and the ability to let go of an outcome is as challenging as the rockiest, tree-rooted trails.

Letting go in life is always a work in progress. Just when we've relaxed our grip on one element, we find our fingers curled tightly around another.

August 13

. . . practice imperfect

Practice letting go. Know that practice will never make perfect. Practice moves toward the grace of excellence.

August 14

. . . content, not complacent

When I was into my forties, my father pointed out to me that I was in a bit of a bind. I was never quite satisfied with what I'd made of myself. Every time I achieved something I'd been working toward, I moved the goal posts farther out.

I bet you're familiar with that maneuver.

Goal posts support our intentions. We will keep moving them out. What my father was pointing out was my tendency to spend too little time enjoying the goal posts as I passed them. I confused complacency with being content.

Now I try to make a point to savor success as it comes and use the contentment as fuel for the next challenge.

Wow—I ran 30K over mountains. I'd like to go faster, but still . . . *wow*.

August 15

. . . new chapters

Kimberly knows about moving goal posts. When she moved to Rwanda, she quit what, to all appearances, was a very successful life. She built herself a new successful life in Kigali, but

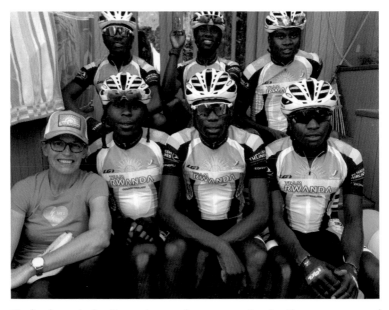

Kimberly with the Rwandan cycling team. *Credit: Photo courtesy of Kimberly*

after eight years, it was time to move the goal posts. Local Rwandans needed to take over the cycling team.

She's had practice at making radical change. She knows she can do it. Even if the change feels uncomfortable in these early days. Her personal mission guides her: "To build and enliven and inspire the unlocked and unlimited potential for greatness in all people."

She and her husband have since moved to his family's ranch in a remote, mountainous part of Wyoming. They are building a place of refuge. Kimberly has a dream of creating her own *bigger table* (taking a page out of John Pavlovitz's book of the same name). Her table will be, as she says, "Inclusive, diverse, a place where we can have differences of opinion and respect each other, a place of truth and respect."

All this, plus the opportunity to be active and outdoors in the mountains—it sounds like an incredible place to be.

August 16

. . . around then over

Where I mountain bike in the Sierra is a "School of Rocks." I struggle to learn how to maneuver around particular rocks, or clusters, over successive summers. Finally I'll find the key, which unlocks the two-wheeled move. What happens next is the curious thing. Often, I then transition from the complicated navigation *around*, which I've mastered at long last, to just riding right *over* the rocks, which is ultimately easier.

I could not have ridden straight over the rocks as an opening gambit. I needed to develop the skill and confidence by first riding around. Only then could I trust my ability to ride over.

There are times we need to do things the hard way to gain the confidence to do those same things the easy way.

August 17

. . . no force, just flow

The Headmistress of the School of Rocks was maybe the size of an upholstered footstool (a rock I will never go over . . . I don't think). She was the first teacher to show me the key, which I use to this day to unlock the puzzle of many rocks. The Headmistress menaced me for three summers. The trail winds around her in a sharp-ish turn, flanked by thick, tie-your-bike-up mountain shrubbery. I always balked at the last minute, and put a steadying foot down. Then one day, I approached my rock-nemesis with more calm than usual. What was the worst that could happen? A tumble in the bushes? A chain ring in my calf? Been there. Done that. I glanced at The Headmistress. Every other day, I stared in dread, but this day my eyes were friendly. The rock seemed to soften, the path to widen. Around I went. No force. Just flow.

I felt my energy slow down. Not sapped or diminished; rather, my energy gathered inward, moving toward my center, that place of balance, which can never be achieved through pushy frustration.

That beautiful zenergy is followed, of course, by the all-important *woohoos* of delight and a mini-party on the bike with helmet-loads of imaginary glitter-confetti.

The physical feeling of gathering energy inward, practiced over and over, dials in at a cellular level, and slowly, but surely, nourishes the rest of our life.

August 18

. . . not going over every day

Of course, my progress (on the bike and in life) is not a straight line. The morning after writing about The Headmistress, I approached a small-ish boulder from below and, in an excess of confidence, instead of going around, I tried to ride right up the side and over. Well, that didn't work. As I write this, the next day, I'm nursing quite a few scrapes and bruises and am very thankful for my helmet.

A few hours later, I thought—maybe I just need to gear down sooner and increase my speed; take a better run at it.

August 19

. . . over she goes

The next time I rode the new-nemesis boulder's trail, I decided definitively that I was going to ride *around*. When the big rock came into view, my heart jumped like a wild woman and then settled. I geared down, gathered inward, revved up, pedaled like crazy, and suddenly I was heading *over*. My bike

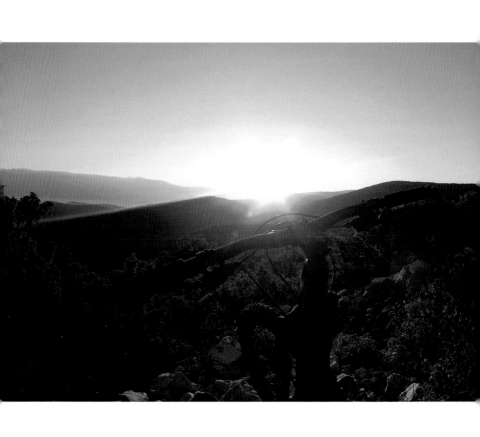

paused on top (as if to say, "Look where I am!"). I breathed out. Don't clench. Over she goes.

Break out the glitter-confetti!

You'd think that conquering obstacles would get old. It doesn't.

August 20

. . . bike flight

I've gotten so bold on Will, after my little series of successes, that I finish my mountain bike rides no-handed (remember when I figured out how to ride no-handed back in April?).

When I come off the trail, there's a final short stretch on paved road to get home. I stretch out my arms and pretend I'm flying.

Zing! Does. Not. Get. Old.

August 21

. . . gentle aggression

I went mountain biking the day after that grueling 30K race in the mountains. I was spinning out my legs, or so the wisdom goes. Maneuvering through some challenging sections, I realized that not only was I riding easier, I was riding faster. Too tired to spend all the effort of being fearful and braking, I was letting the bike go more. Often I feel aggressive when I'm mountain biking, as if I'm attacking the hard parts. This day, I was gentle on the bike and the obstacles ceded.

So often, being on my mountain bike is an object lesson in how to live. More trust. Less fear. More ease. Less fight.

August 22

. . . Susan B. Anthony cycled

"Bicycling has done more to emancipate women than any one thing in the world . . . A woman awheel is the picture of untrammeled womanhood."
—Susan B. Anthony

A suffragist who fought for women's right to vote, Susan B. wrote that in 1896, in her publication, *Revolution*.

Whether or not you cycle, we are untrammeled women.

August 23

. . . velocipede

When Susan B. wrote about bicycling, she was jumping into a fray that had been going on for some time. Her fellow suffragist, Frances Willard, had written an article, "How I Learned to Ride the Bicycle," in 1895, which provoked outrage. *Among other women*! Women who believed that the sexes must maintain their respective dependent and protective positions, else they would lose interest in one another. "When a lady velocipedes, she destroys all this kind of subtle interest," one editorial said.

Exercising our citizenship in the world is not a subtle business.

August 24

. . . being outdoors is fun, I promise

The University of North Carolina has made personal fitness and wellness courses required for every student. No matter who you are, you at least have to take a walking class, or walk to jog, or yoga or Pilates. Within the next academic year, UNC's Wilmington campus will have beach walking. Sign me up.

AmberLynn teaches many of the personal fitness classes and, as she says, "It blows my mind how many students would rather stay inside on the 1/8th mile track than go outdoors." The students don't want to sweat, or the outdoors just seems more daunting. Once they get outside, most agree it's more fun.

I'm from the school of pretty-much-any-sport-is-better-outdoors. It's been heartening to see a number of studies confirm the extra benefits of being in nature—on the beach, amidst trees or fields, on a river or lake, or mountains.

Remember when your parents told you to go outside and play? They were right.

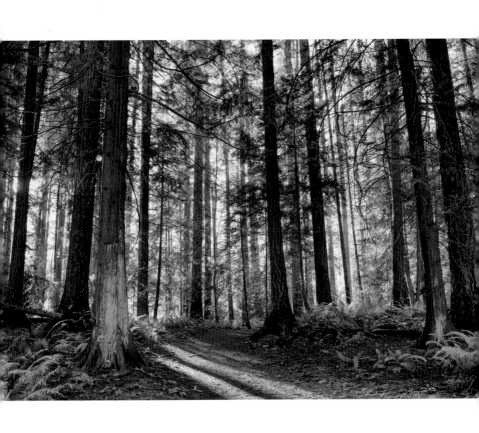

August 25

. . . between pine trees

"Between every two pine trees there is a door leading to a new way of life."

—John Muir

The Scottish-American naturalist and mountaineer captures the essence of why I love to be out on the trails. Outdoors, in the elements in any season, is where we can get our daily dose of the ineffable.

August 26

. . . a commitment to health

AmberLynn didn't grow up in an outdoor fitness environment. When she was in high school she looked around her family and community and saw a lot of people who were neglecting their physical wellbeing. So, she made a choice to take care of her health. She has a master's in exercise science and she will not put away her dream of completing a PhD. In the meantime, she's undertaken the hard work of motivating classes full of mostly unwilling participants to move. That takes commitment and a strong sense of purpose.

August 27

. . . just say it—I am an athlete

AmberLynn and her long-time training partner have been building up their running together. From 5K to 8K to 10K, now they're aiming at a 15K. Her partner is fleet enough that she often places in her age group, yet she won't call herself an athlete. AmberLynn points out that men who haven't played football (or done much of anything athletic since high school) will still call themselves athletes, whereas women are hesitant to claim the word, even when they are training and competing on a regular basis.

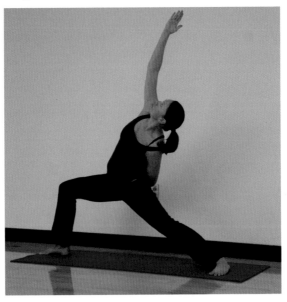

AmberLynn in warrior pose. *Credit: Photo courtesy of AmberLynn*

AmberLynn is encouraging her running partner to try the word on for size: "Instead of telling people you're a stay-at-home mom, tell them you're a runner."

Women are comfortable with all the relational descriptors—wife, mother, daughter, sister—but we need to get better claiming our individual achievements.

Let's say it together: I am an athlete.

August 28

. . . reuniting our bodies and our selves

"As women, we often separate our physical selves from the rest of our lives," athlete and activist artist Leslie says. "At least that was true with my generation. When we find the balance of being in our bodies, we end up more centered."

Yes we do.

August 29

. . . radical love

"One of the most radical things women can do is to love their body."

—Eve Ensler

Be radical.

August 30

. . . work out because you love your body

"Work out because you love your body, not because you hate it."

—Samantha Brennan and Tracy Isaacs

Words we can live by from their book, *Fit at Mid-Life: A Feminist Fitness Journey.*

August 31

. . . summer camp

On this last day of the official summer months, one of the highlights of my childhood summers comes to mind.

I remember my father leaving me at overnight summer camp for the first time. He took a picture of me right before he left. I was twelve, in shorts and a t-shirt, all long skinny arms and legs. I looked breakable, but I stayed brave until my father was gone. Then I hid behind my cabin to cry, sick for home. Maybe I had a premonition, because that co-ed camp experience was horrible and I never went back. The next year my parents sent me to an all-girls camp that my mother and her mother had gone to. I ended up going there for many summers and loved it. I have vivid memories of practicing canoe strokes out in the middle of the lake alone. Camp was one of the formative experiences in my life. I have no memory of my first moments at GBC. I was probably homesick then, too, but the feeling was quickly forgotten, replaced by the joy of getting to be me in all my girl strength.

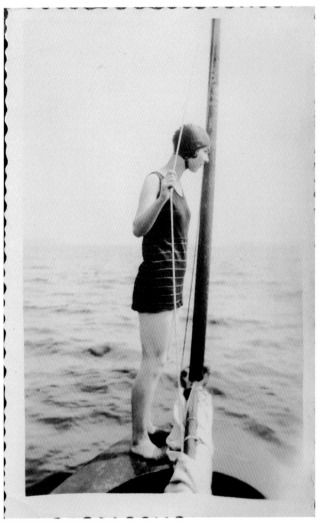

Grandnan at Glen Bernard Camp, 1929. *Credit: Photo courtesy of the author*

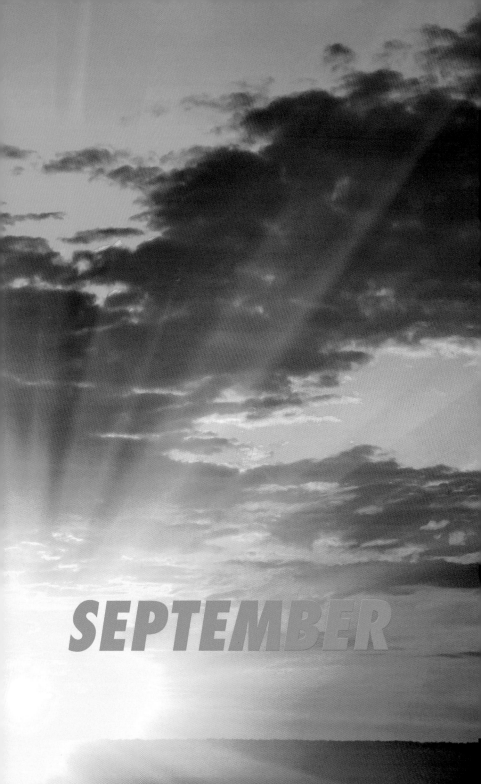

SEPTEMBER

September 1

. . . a morning person

Even now, at quite a distance from my last eraser-scented, back-to-school year, I think about buying a new pencil case and waking up a little earlier when September rolls around.

Growing up in my family, I didn't seem like a morning person, because my father's idea of *morning* was 5:00 a.m. On Sundays, he would play marching bands at top volume starting at about 7:30 a.m. Because why in the world would anyone want to sleep later? I envy teenagers who sleep until noon. Maybe if I'd had the practice when I was young, I'd be able to do it now. Instead, a big sleep-in generally only takes me to 8:30 a.m., at best.

I've run at all different times of the day and evening, but my favorite time of all is probably 7:30 a.m. on a weekday—before breakfast, decadently late by my father's standards, but not so luxurious as to make me feel like a dilettante. It's hard to shake what you grew up with.

What's your favored hour for a workout? Do you experiment?

September 2

. . . trigger an avalanche in your mind and body

It's time to go for your run. The alarm just went off. Do you snooze and skip your run, or do you get up? If you don't need more sleep, get up. Not only will you feel better for making that first right decision, you'll set off a little avalanche of neuropsychological and neurobiological goodness in your body.

The positive cascade of emotions you trigger when you do what you intend releases dopamine (responsible for alertness). This activates circuits that fire other neurotransmitters, which in turn increases production of things like serotonin (for focus) and norepinephrine (for wellbeing). Meanwhile, cortisol, which you need when you're stressed, takes a snooze. Brain Derived Neurotrophic Factor (BDNF) can do its work without cortisol interfering. BDNF is responsible for neurogenesis: that's the generation of new brain cells, that's your brain growing.

By the way, BDNF is also produced when we exercise intensely. By sticking to your workout (and not stressing out on judgment or blame for sleeping in), you've doubled your brain/body benefit, just like that.

Thank you science for getting us out of bed.

September 3

... high school

I hope you enjoyed high school more than I did. Quite often, when I'm running, I'll think about that girl, filled to the brim with self-doubt, struggling to find her place in the world. I wish I could have taken her on a run up a mountain trail and shown her what she was going to be capable of.

September 4

... inherited self-image

Kim inherited her poor self-image from her mother, a woman who walked compulsively to manage her constant worrying. When her mother took her shopping for clothes when Kim was a child, she would loudly ask for size large, in a tone designed to shame her daughter.

From softball to dancing, Kim believed that she was terrible at any activity she tried to do with her body. In university she was an egghead (well, she still is, as a professor of theatre studies), but she also discovered rowing.

The sport showed her that she was strong. Sadly, her rowing coach focused all his attention on the blonde, ponytailed members of the team. Kim never had the opportunity to develop her talent to the fullest.

More years passed, while Kim's psyche swam in a soup of anxiety much like her mother's. Until one day, shopping for a pair of trousers at the Gap, she realized that she needed another size up. She could almost hear her mother's voice asking for the larger size.

In that dressing room, Kim made a decision to break with the self-image her mother had passed down to her. Of course, transcending a lifetime of negativity didn't happen in the time it took to leave the store, but Kim had started the work.

To change we need to be aware and intentional.

September 5

. . . loving herself on the bike

After setting her intention in that dressing room, Kim started running and swimming and lifting. When ankylosing spondylitis—a potentially crippling arthritis of the spine—sidelined her running, she fell into road biking, almost by accident. She was good at it. This time she found a coach who paid attention to her. She wasn't just strong; she was courageous.

"I can be a version of myself I love. I have a freedom on the bike that I can't have elsewhere in my life. Freedom from anxiety."

Kim says that she's been "properly sporty" for more than fifteen years.

"If I ever went on *RuPaul's Drag Race*, I would dress in a giant inflatable bicycle," Kim says. "Not that I qualify for the show [an uber-campy drag queen contest], obviously, but still, I feel like I've found my drag identity."

Our sports have the power to expand our identities in the most unexpected ways.

September 6

. . . to be more capacious in the world

Cycling taught Kim to be, as she says, "More capacious in the world." Being in a pack on the bike, in immediate relationship with the road and everything around her—the animals, the other riders, pedestrians, drivers—demanded her presence in a new way.

Her expanded sense of the world opened her to a new relationship with her work. She grew up thinking she had to do things that made people proud of her. Now she knows there's much more to life than striving for the gold star. Instead, she thinks about how she wants her life to be. She has more energy for the daily professional struggle of getting people to care about theatre.

September 7

. . . love to sweat

To expand our presence in the world involves sweat. Not just metaphorical sweat, but the real kind that runs in your eyes. I love the feeling of a good, big sweat in a workout. The

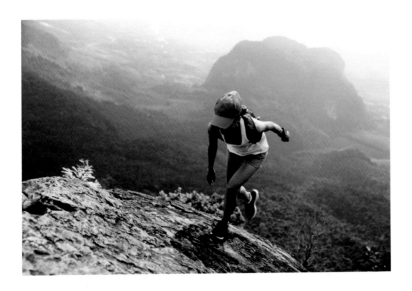

cleanse feels physical, mental and emotional. Another thing I love about a sweaty workout is that it's allowed. Sure, there are probably people who still think that a lady doesn't sweat.

Those people live under the rocks we run and ride and ski and hike and climb over.

September 8

. . . sweat confession

I said that bit about people who think women don't sweat with great bravado. But the truth is that when I'm not working out, I also sweat—a lot. This is something I haven't generally told people about. Most of the time, I can't wear colored tops, not anything except black, and sometimes white. In any other color, I usually end up with my arms pinned to my sides at some point during the day, waiting for the big circle of sweat under my arms to dry, which, of course, it can't, because I have my arms clamped down.

When I worked as a lawyer, I would try to wear colored silk blouses under my suit jackets, but then I couldn't take off my jacket. The result was that I often looked unnecessarily formal, not to mention that I was often hot, compounding the original challenge.

Eventually I gave up on trying to wear colors. No antiperspirant ever worked. I thought fleetingly about having my sweat glands removed under my arms. Is that even possible? Where does the sweat go then?

I'd like to say that being an athlete has helped me overcome my embarrassment about what I perceive as my excessive sweating. But it hasn't. I think it's one of the reasons I extra love my sweaty workouts. No shame in a good sweat there.

September 9

. . . physical therapy

I went for a course of treatment by a physical therapist who was somewhat non-traditional. One of the techniques he used was dry needling, a version of acupuncture that applies the needle directly to the affected area, instead of using the lines of energy in our body, as traditional acupuncture does. He told me that he'd never encountered anyone who sweated as instantaneously and as profusely as I did. He laughed (nicely) at my feet, which would drip as soon as he started applying needles.

All these years I've worked really hard to hide my sweat "problem," accommodating for it in my wardrobe, not talking about it, and so on. And here I was a source of fascination. Yet his calling attention to my sweat was liberating. I laughed with him about my feet, about the drops of sweat that in fact beaded anywhere he put a needle on my body. In his office, this source of shame wasn't one anymore. My body, he told me, was just hyper efficient. That sounded like a good thing. I didn't need to be ashamed of my sweat.

September 10

. . . sweat fears

At the vision quest I did in New Mexico, there was a woman in her fifties who had never been in a relationship with anyone for more than a one-night stand. She believed that that was partially because she smelled bad (she didn't!). Of course, there were other root causes for her great fear of intimacy. There always are. But, as someone who has struggled with her own sweat issues, I felt a kinship grief for what she'd lost.

When I'd first met her, I'd thought, *Oh I have nothing in common with her.* Only to then discover that we shared intimate fears.

September 11

. . . a pause for reflection

On September 11, 2001, I went for my regular Tuesday morning run with my longtime running partner. The morning was gorgeous. The sky was as blue as it gets in Central Park. The air had the first hints of that fall freshness.

This is a day to reflect on the delusion that we are separate. There is no *us and them*.

We are.

September 12

. . . let your body show you

We women are prone to finding fault with our bodies, to engaging in down-talk.

Every time Kim encounters a new woman in her cycling group who is sure she isn't strong enough to be at the front of the pack, she takes the woman under her wing. Kim wants to share the benefits cycling has offered her. She takes the time to show her comrade women cyclists how to ride at the front and how to recuperate. Most importantly, she tells the women, "Trust your body in its strength and then take some leaps and let your body show you what you can do."

September 13

. . . take your own breath away

As confident as she is of her body on the bike, Kim didn't start buying lingerie until her early forties.

As girls (and women, too), we get a lot of messages that tell us our body is not good enough, that it needs to be disciplined, slimmed down, and forced into a certain look. Worse, we women are the prime conspirators in this shaming. Kim has certainly felt this pressure for a long time and the easy-1-2-3 of the *love yourself* message that proliferates practically everywhere feels empty to her.

Take lingerie shopping, which Kim waited a long time to do. Does even the contemplation of the excursion set off alarm bells in your head? If not, lucky you! I buy the majority of my bras and underwear online. Brick and mortar lingerie stores are reserved for days I feel extra good about myself, happy not to have cleavage to worry about when I'm running.

Kim found one of those rare lingerie stores whose mission is to find something a woman feels good in, that's comfortable (I know, how novel, right?), and that she wants. The slogan at Stole My Heart (that's the store, which is in Toronto) is, "Take your own breath away."

That should be a slogan for a lot more in life.

September 14

... race shirts

I wonder what would happen if we worked out wearing a shirt that said, "Take Your Own Breath Away."

Thinking about this reminds me of Dr. Masaru Emoto's experiments with water and the power of thoughts and words. The Emoto Peace Project showed that when kind words were spoken (or even taped!) to a glass of water, the water would then freeze into beautiful patterns, whereas harsh words and thoughts would turn the same water into ugly ice crystals. The movie *What the Bleep Do We Know?* is built on this same idea. Emoto's ideas may seem cockamamie and refutable. Personally, I not only accept the results, I'm inspired.

How about race T-shirts from events we participated in? We are carrying the event's competitive energy and sense of accomplishment with us on the road (kind words to water, after all, our bodies are 90 percent water). The shirt is a personal fairy on our shoulders, reminding us that we can do it. We've done it before.

September 15

... running topless

I always wear a shirt when I'm running, no matter how hot

it gets. Sure, I say it's for protection from the sun, but really it's because I'm self-conscious about how I look in only a running bra.

In 2014, I was home visiting my parents and went out for a run. It was a beautiful September morning. A bit overcast, some humidity, but one of those first cooling weather days. I was overdressed in my long-sleeved shirt. Halfway into the run I was into that push-up-my-sleeves-every-ten-steps mode. It would have been much easier just to take off my shirt. But I don't, so I didn't.

I kept running and heating up. I was thinking about the conversation I'd had with my father before I left for the run. It was about assisted suicide, something he was contemplating as he headed into weeks of radiation for a third, aggressive recurrence of melanoma. I supported his decision without any qualms. Our conversation was matter of fact, in our family way, which made it all the more surreal. I needed the run to bring me back to earth, into my body, to let my heart feel, to allow space for the enormous sadness.

The air was exquisite. As I thought about my father maybe not being around, I took off my shirt. How I looked without my shirt on didn't matter. I was alive and well, and that was all that mattered.

September 16

... teardrop

With my shirt off, the light chill on my stomach felt like a childhood memory of my mother blowing on my soft baby tummy. Had my mother actually done that? Or was I tapping into the collective memory of all the babies whose mothers and fathers had blown on their tummies?

On that September morning run, the air and my skin merged, sweat and humidity mingling, as if I were suspended inside a teardrop, the breath of the universe tickling my skin, comforting me.

September 17

. . . bed-and-breakfast conversation

My father liked nothing better than to dive into a conversation with strangers. I, on the other hand, get nervous about conversations with new people. Yet, when I get over myself, often I am gifted something beautiful in the enforced conversation. Here's one.

My partner and I were on a one-night romantic getaway in a bed-and-breakfast in Nevada City. The owner struck up a conversation with us at breakfast. He pulled an object from his pocket and declared that it was the morning mystery. At first, I felt annoyed. I wanted breakfast, not guessing games.

The object he showed us was the size of a small tree branch, an inch or so in diameter and three or four inches long. The surface was a pale pebbly grey, rough to the touch, like rugged cement. The object looked as if it might have been part of a larger object. The ends were sheared smooth, revealing a darker grey, glassy surface, ringed by paler shades.

We guessed something from the sea. It had a coral quality.

No. A fossilized tree branch, because it had an enchanted forest look. No. We gave up.

"Fulgurite," our host declared.

"How do you spell that?" I asked.

I already knew I was going to look the word up later. That word alone dazzled me. But what was it?

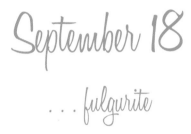

September 18

. . . fulgurite

"Petrified lightning," he continued. "It forms when lightning strikes sand. This came from the desert. It was part of a much larger piece, three branches total and about ten feet at its longest."

I imagined an entire upside-down forest of petrified lightning, hidden from view, deep in the desert. A moment captured for all eternity; the ultimate 3D photograph, a burst of light and energy made solid. I rest my mind against the image sometimes, watching the lightning strike and the earth transform.

September 19

. . . giving up on a run

Our whole short getaway to Nevada City might have been a story of frustration, but instead it bestowed us with gifts of unexpected beauty. Before the fulgurite, there was the run the day before. We'd planned twenty miles, with six-thousand feet of elevation gain. We had three liters of water for the two of us. Oh, and it was 95 degrees.

I hate giving up on a run. In this, I'm like a dog with a chew toy—I won't let go. But after four and a half hours and fifteen miles, I had to admit that it was time to give up. The road where we pulled out was un-trafficked. How were we going to find a ride? The first couple of side roads led off into dense and menacing woods. Finally, we saw a house set back in the trees. At the gate, a tiny rock was painted with the words "inquire about our guest cabin." Was the cabin referred to the structure with the tin-sheet roof, caving-in walls and no door, set some twenty-five feet from the house? Was the sign ironic? And how about the large empty dog cage?

This run was not turning out as anticipated.

September 20

. . . Ruby

I walked toward the house with trepidation. No dog in sight. Just two little cats, heads popping up and then bounding away, tails pointed skyward. A woman in her mid-fifties answered the rickety screen door with a friendly smile. She offered her phone—a landline—to call into Nevada City for a taxi. She went back to cutting hearts out of a spot-patterned bed sheet. I asked after the dog and she told me he had died.

But then the women led me into her bedroom. There, lounging and snorting at the end of the bed, on her own crib mattress (complete with sheets and extra bolster pillows) was Ruby, a 160-pound Vietnamese potbelly pig. Seventeen years old, arthritic and ailing, Ruby was a former service pig. She had visited hospices, hospitals, and schools in her prime and had sported the pig-fashions of the day. I petted Ruby and looked at her baby book, which included a younger Ruby in a Sugar Plum Fairy outfit.

Inside myself, I felt a fresh flow of energy, as my internal rhythm re-calibrated from the truncated exertion of the run to this new, unlooked for experience, finding the adjusted harmony in the day. We didn't force the run. We flowed around the challenges, to find the most natural course for that day.

September 21

. . . running to Dyckman

So many days bring me versions of fulgurite and Ruby. One day my partner and I decided to run up to the northern tip of Manhattan, about eight miles from our apartment. We wanted to check out a recently opened nature trail. We planned to then have lunch at the new restaurant at the Dyckman docks, where only a few short years before there had been nothing.

The day was warm and sunny, the running comfortable. My partner told me about some new things he'd learned about Gingko trees in the city, from a book he'd come across by chance, only to then discover it had been written by someone he had known twenty years ago when he'd lived on a boat on the Hudson River by Riverside Park. What a coincidence. Then, to compound the coincidence, less than ten minutes later we ran into the author on the new nature trail. My partner hadn't seen her for at least a decade. We were infused with that feeling of magical alignment the universe delivers now and then.

September 22

. . . the romance of hazard

At the restaurant, the lobster rolls and fries were decadent and delicious; and other than our high-performance-wicking-clothed selves, the crowd looked like it was a fashion shoot for a Jazz Age brunch—men wore straw hats with ribbon bands and two-toned shoes, women poured into their dresses like saltwater taffy, perched on their fruit-colored heels. Our table looked out at the river and the unspoiled green of Palisades Park across the water. Manhattan was hidden around a bend in the river. It was as if we had run right out of the dirty, crowded city into a genteel town where people had gardens and wrap-around porches.

Deep into my forties and two decades into our relationship, I got the giggles. The confluence of circumstances felt right and uniquely romantic to our relationship, which had started in running clothes at a nice restaurant.

September 23

. . . poetry everywhere

That day at Dyckman felt like poetry. Everywhere we look an experience juxtaposes with a new reality and we can find a fresh rhyme, an unexpected rhythm. We are implicated in the universe's grace.

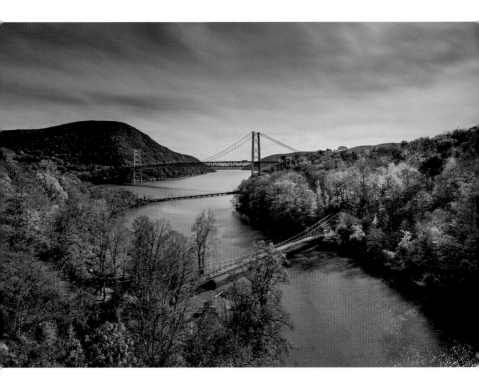

September 24

. . . being a statistic.

One of my favorite poems is by Wislawa Szymborska, titled (at least in one of my translated editions): "A Contribution to Statistics." The poem enumerates a starkly beautiful list of probabilities. Here are two of my favorites:

Out of a hundred people

[. . .]

Those who always know better
—fifty-two

doubting every step
—nearly all the rest

We all live in the balance between *I'm sure* and *I doubt*.

September 25

. . . the Goal of Everything

After reading one of my favorite poems, I can't help thinking about the way we set goals. How they give us a sense of purpose in the midst of much doubt.

Every goal we set—and every goal we don't—relates to what physicists might call the Goal of Everything (GOE). Physicists have many theories about the universe, which often compete with and contradict one another. A physicist's dream is to find a unifying theory. This Theory of Everything (TOE) would marry quantum physics and general relativity. In our personal lives, the GOE is the goal that ties all our other goals together, that which underpins everything we do. It is the how and why of our persistence.

The GOE is to be happy. We fill our happy when we bring more happiness into the world. Fulfilled.

September 26

... four sublime states

Loving-kindness (or just plain love), compassion, joy, and equanimity are called the four sublime states in Buddhist thinking. Taken together, I don't think we can do better than defining the constituent elements of the *happy* we want to be and the happiness we want to bring into the world.

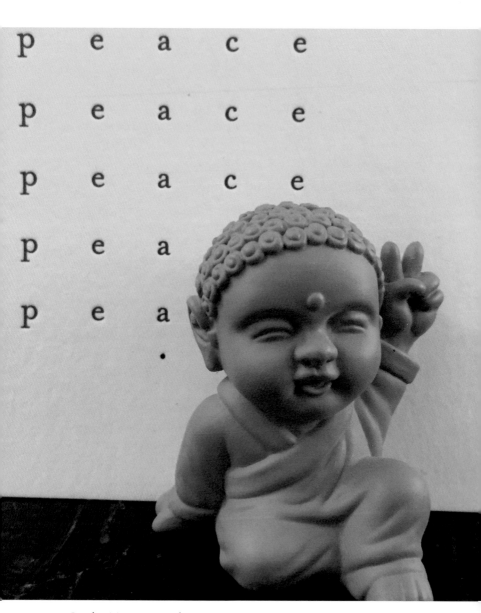

Credit: Mina Samuels

September 27

. . . equanimous

I wasn't always sold on equanimity as an essential contributor to the sublime states. Who wants to be equanimous? It sounds too much like squamous—those are the cells on the skin where cancers occur—for comfort. What's sublime about being even and balanced all the time? Where's the fun in that? At a silent meditation retreat, I started crying uncontrollably at the thought that true equanimity would deprive me of those sudden, random, surprise moments of unbridled joy—when you see a tree in full fall foliage; when, as the song goes, a snowflake sticks to your eyelash.

September 28

. . . equanimity

Finally a wise person explained to me that equanimity wasn't about negating the upside. Equanimity is not a sourpuss telling me to stop having fun and to laugh more quietly. Rather, it is about not stressing the downside so much and not wrecking the upside by grabbing at it too hard. The grand theatricality of a major meltdown used to feel to me like living fully. Now it feels like a self-destructive waste of time. I'm starting to see how equanimity can be a pretty good gig—abundant joy and smaller portions of drama and other self-generated suffering.

September 29

. . . the process is the goal

What's interesting about the GOE and the four sublime states is that they are all about process, not about outcome. That's how we should approach all our goals. Do you want to be happier tomorrow? Enjoy today first. Want to be the boss? Love the job you do now, on your way to the corner office. Training for a race? Be sure that you enjoy the months of running leading up to the race, instead of focusing on the race time you're aiming for. Chances are high that your race will go better if you are thinking less about a time goal and more about enjoying the process.

Once again, science has our back on this one. Studies find that people persist better when they are focusing on the *process* of exercise itself vs. the *instrumental goals* of a workout (running a certain speed, losing a certain amount of weight).

Love your run and the race performance will take care of itself, or not. If it doesn't conform to expectations, so what? Don't resent the disappointment. If the training is happy, you will want to try again.

September 30

. . . meditation is a process, too

This seems like a good time to point out that this whole *process* vs. *instrumental goal* focus applies to our time meditating. I am often guilty of trying to be instrumental with my meditation practice. I'll meditate for the specific goal of de-stressing or finding calm before a challenge.

Over the years, I've noticed that after a more instrumental-goal-focused meditation (say, I want to quiet my mind), I'm more prone to be short-tempered afterward. Whereas when I meditate for no reason, simply to engage in the process, then I am more likely to feel lighter afterward.

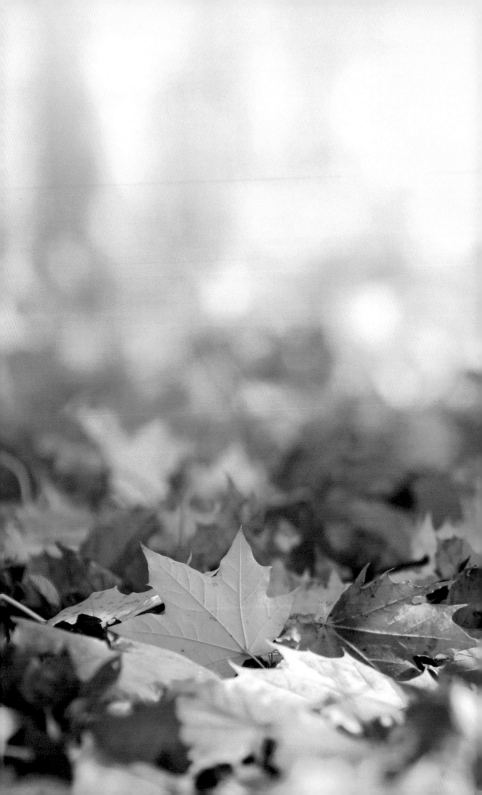

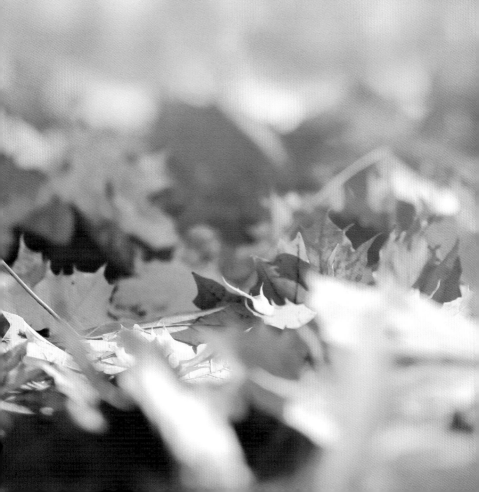

OCTOBER

October 1

. . . apples

I grew up spending holiday weekends at my grandparents' apple farm. We grandchildren would be set loose upon the orchard to play and summoned back for meals by the distant sound of a ringing gong. We would visit the sand dunes, a little hill of soil that had eroded down to fine sand, and the big woods and the medium woods. These were small, forested areas that bordered the edges of the orchard. Not to be confused with the baby woods, which consisted of five tall pines clustered in a circle in the middle of the orchard.

Come autumn, we ate apples right off the tree. The tartness. The crunchiness. The sweetness. I would eat until I got

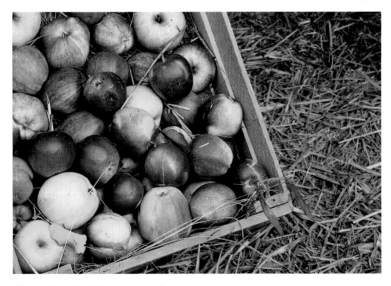

Photo Credit: Mina Samuels

a stomachache and the fruity acid burned the inside of my mouth.

The orchard is where I first fell in love with the outdoors.

October 2

. . . taking the plunge

One time I paid money for the opportunity to plunge into a pool of icy water and swim under a wall that divided the pool in half. I don't just mean ice cold. I mean water thick with a deep layer of floating ice cubes better suited to the inside of a martini shaker. When I, in my panic, tried to surface, it felt as if the ice cubes were pressing down on top of me.

I was participating in a Mt. Snow, Vermont iteration of the obstacle course race phenomenon—a Tough Mudder.

This particular event had more than thirty obstacles. In addition to the dumpster ice bath, there were cables and monkey bars and balance beams over heart-stoppingly icy water. Jumping off ledges (into icy water). Running through smoke. Jumping over fires. Scaling walls. Crawling on your belly under barbed or live electrical wire or through culverts. Oh, and ten miles of mountain running, with a bonus of deep mud and hidden rocks.

This is not a traditional race. The environment prizes collaboration over speed, and a good attitude over finish time. The event is about facing down your fears and staying strong in the jaws of exhaustion . . . and having fun (lest we forget)!

I forgot.

October 3

. . . obstacles for their own sake

I am a good swimmer, but fearful of cold water. I'm not a fan of that feeling of suffocation that sets in when I'm immersed in too-cold water. I'm sure with training, I could learn, if not to love, then not to fear that feeling. But how unpleasant would all that training be, and to what end?

I know I can plunge into icy water when necessary. The question is, why would I?

You already know that I think sports are one of the most efficacious ways to train in a microcosm of life's challenges and get invaluable glimpses into how much more we are capable of. It's a good thing to face our fears. In so doing we strengthen our spirit (and possibly our bodies). If we never challenge ourselves (which necessarily involves facing fear— of a concrete thing, like cold water, or of a less tangible thing, like failure), then we will cease to grow. True engagement in

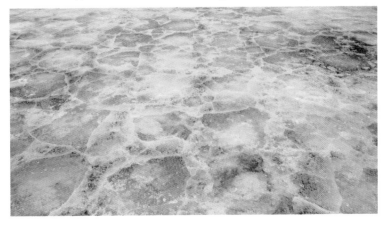

the world demands our willingness, even our desire, to greet and, yes, seek out challenges.

The question the Tough Mudder posed was, are these the right challenges for me? No. I did not enjoy the process and the instrumental goal felt artificial.

We don't always have to add to our list of challenges. We can delete. Leaves more room for loving the process of what we want to do.

October 4

. . . life is a Tough Mudder

I'm often sleepless before an ultra-marathon, terrified I can't finish or that I'll hurt myself on the mountain or that the pain in general might be too much. I also thrive on that fear and am all the more thrilled when I finish. There were many at the Tough Mudder who loved the challenges and derived huge pleasure from the whole event. My compatriot throughout the event was an energetic, inspiring woman. The whole group I participated with was full of wonderful spirits. I am glad I participated.

The intense, externally generated focus forced me to be in that much ballyhooed *moment* we are often counseled to live in: when we are fully committed to an activity; when we have reached the point of casting aside self-doubt and fear; when we still the chatter in our mind; when we actually *just do it*; and when we glory in the feeling of our bodies in motion. I've proved to myself I can do it. Once was enough.

I thought I would love the Tough Mudder. But it felt like

obstacles for their own sake. Whereas running up a mountain feels purposeful. Everyone is different. Life is its own Tough Mudder every day.

Take on the extracurricular challenges that are joyful. There's no reason to put more unpleasant obstacles in your path.

October 5

. . . Tough Mudder meditation

A couple of months before the Tough Mudder, I went on my first silent meditation retreat. It was one week long. In addition to no talking, we were also asked not to read, write, listen to music, watch movies or television, or use a computer. I had only the inside of my mind—and a daily dharma talk— for company. I didn't even run. Instead I went for a vigorous walk every day.

An extended period of silence and meditation reaches toward the same goals as the Tough Mudder, but from the opposite vantage point—one of stillness and an internally generated focus. Generating the mindfulness that enables me to catch glimpses, to touch, even briefly, the radiant expansiveness of a clear mind, is at least as challenging as jumping in an ice bath. Seven days alone with the contents of my head and I sometimes felt like my mind and I were barely on speaking terms. I was knee-deep in muck, just as surely as I had been running up Mt. Snow. But sometimes, for the blink of an eye, a pause occurred between the thoughts, the mud settled, and there, for an instant, was clarity; a feeling like turning myself inside out and immersing myself in a mild effervescence.

October 6

... counting ten breaths

There's a particular hill on my trail running routes that's shallow enough I can really push up the hill on a good day. Often to focus my mind (taking a leaf out of the meditation playbook) I count to ten as I'm running that hill. With each outbreath I'll think, *One, breathe, two, breathe, three*, and so on. On a good day I'll mostly catch myself before I think, *Eleven*. On a distracted day, I'll find that I've hit nineteen, having forgotten my ten-count mantra in the time it took to count.

You can guess which days I'm running faster, smoother, stronger.

October 7

... counting to ten only works for so long

So why don't I just count to ten for my whole run? On every hill, from the shallowest to the steepest?

Because.

I can't do the technique for extended periods of time. Here's the bad news—focusing intensely, but calmly, is hard to do for long stretches. Our minds wander. I forget that I'm counting. I stop counting. Here's the good news—I've discovered that I can focus for longer, when I practice. I do best with this breathing technique on my original ten-breath-hill. That's where I've practiced it the most. It feels natural. I can and do extend the practice to other hills (or flats or downhills), but none feel as simple.

I should practice more. But sometimes, I just want to run and I don't care if it's fast or focused.

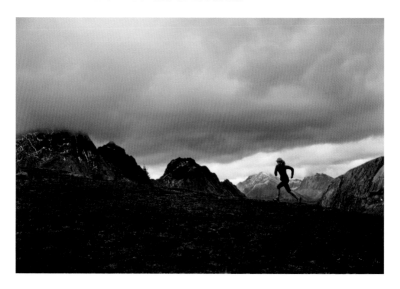

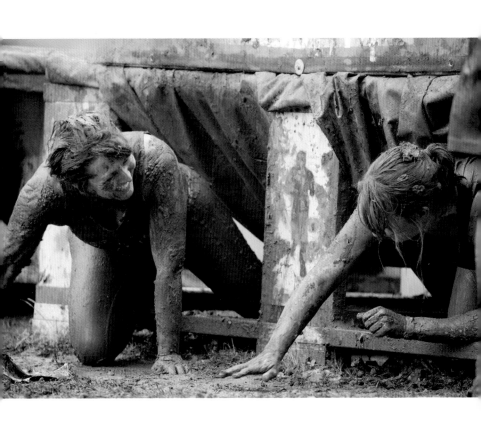

October 8

. . . unlocking an extra piece

Tough Mudder didn't change my life, but obstacle races have certainly changed others'. That's why we need to keep trying new things to see what works for us. Today and tomorrow feature two women whose lives were catalyzed.

Margaret believes the Spartan experience (another obstacle race) "helps unlock an extra piece of ourselves." In her case, a month before her twenty-ninth birthday in 2010, she quit her day job working in admissions and college placement and coaching to devote herself full-time to the risky proposition of depending on race sponsors, writing her blog *Dirt in Your Skirt*, and helping other women get active. Margaret turned her passion into her profession. She went from weekend warrior to industry professional, by writing books and articles, hosting a podcast, coaching, and giving back to the community.

October 9

. . . more than her share of obstacles

At eighteen years old, Ella Anne got hooked on Spartan races. Considering that she'd had way more than her share of obstacles, there's poetry in that fact. When she was thirteen, a horseback riding accident resulted in a broken back—an injury that was aggravated significantly by a birth defect in which Ella's spine was not connected to her sacrum. Four metal rods and screws and a year and a half later, she was back on her feet and running, even if it was painful (okay, *very* painful). Ella knows from experience that the first thing to break down is the mind, and for her the racing is an opportunity to touch her limits, something she finds "very intriguing," fostering a toughness that will no doubt come in handy as life unfolds. From Spartans she's moved onto many other physical adventures, not to mention that she's now an artist.

October 10

. . . slamming my finger in a door

On my way to yoga class one day, in an effort to stop the front door of my apartment from slamming, I caught my middle finger in the heavy locking mechanism. After I'd picked myself back up, finger throbbing, nail instantly blackened, I continued on my way to yoga. I thought it might distract me from the pain. As if. I bailed out after the first downward dog.

By the next morning the fingernail looked like it was straining against the blue-black swelling beneath the nail. I wondered if it would just pop off. My learning curve being slow, I again thought that going to my swim workout would be a diversion from the pain. As if. There's nothing like the arc of a swim stroke to rush the blood into your fingers, increasing any preexisting pain and swelling. I gave up quickly. One of my swim mates suggested I poke a needle through my fingernail to release the blood blister pressure.

No way was I going to do that. I went to the hospital across the street from the pool. I sat in a busy hall of the emergency ward, watching gurneys pass by and medical staff tend to people with far more pressing needs than my paltry finger injury. After a while, I went home and stuck a needle through my fingernail. The technique worked.

Even small moments of mind over pain remind us that we *can* get through more than we think.

October 11

. . . from active to athlete

When Samantha made the career leap from professor of philosophy to dean of the College of Arts it was, as she says, "not unconnected with my athletic side."

Sam grew up in an environment where girls made a choice—books or sports. You were either on a team or a reluctant student in gym class. She chose books. As an undergraduate, she started bike commuting. "I was active, not an athlete," Sam specifies. Serious cycling found Sam when she was in graduate school. She discovered she was a strong rider. Her sense of accomplishment fed her increasing athleticism.

The physical confidence she has in the world as an athlete now means that she's willing to try new things. She knows what it feels like to master something new. Not only physical activities, like her first foray into downhill skiing at fifty-four, but taking on the new role of dean.

October 12

. . . department meetings in bike gear

Sam's new role is demanding. She has less flexibility. Her days are fully scheduled. Taking an hour or two out of her day to cycle isn't an option anymore. Six months in, she is still negotiating the balance. She's had her first meeting in bike gear, on a day she was running later than expected. Her bike is usually on hand in her office, to give her the best chance at squeezing a ride in.

I used to think of philosophers and academic deans as dusty, tweedy, and usually male. Not anymore.

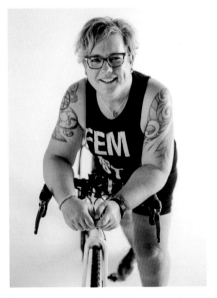

Samantha loves her bike. *Credit: Photo courtesy of Samantha*

October 13

. . . I can, therefore I am

Most of us have read or heard that old Descartes line, "I think, therefore I am." That quote always made me uncomfortable. I couldn't quite put my finger on why, until I read the essay "Look Up From Your Screen," by Nicholas Tampio in *Aeon*. He writes about the created or assumed gap between our minds and our physical bodies in Descartes's words. Well, as athletes we know that our minds and bodies are so interlinked as to be inseparable.

Here's another point of view: in his *Phenomenology of Perception*, French philosopher Maurice Merleau-Ponty wrote, "consciousness is originally not an *I think that*, but rather an *I can*." Turns out we are more Merlau-Pontian than Cartesian.

I *can* run like a girl.

October 14

. . . a true Montreal resident

Letter excerpt to my parents from McGill University on October 14, 1984: *Well Montreal is the same as ever. I even jogged up Mont Royal the other day to feel like a true resident. I almost died when I got to the top.*

October 15

. . . having when-I-was-your-age thoughts

Many miles and years after that first struggle up Mont Royal, doing a new "it" workout *du jour*, the dewy, young instructor was encouraging us to dig deep and overcome the mental barriers preventing us from working to our fullest.

I had a sudden, exasperated thought: *Honey, I've been working out hard since before you were born, and today I don't have that extra-extra-something-something-just-do-it-ness you want me to find.*

Let's face it. Some days our energy is going to stay holed up inside. Good. Take a break. There are days we release our life force into the world and days we gather from the life force others have offered up.

October 16

. . . the years keep passing

I don't want to succumb to cosmetic surgery. It feels like a betrayal; giving in to society's disdain for older women. I think: *Why can't I just be happy with myself as I am? Why can't I embrace the aging process? Why can't I observe the world's gaze turning from me with detachment?*

Do our sports help? Undoubtedly. One of the beauties

(pun intended) of physical effort is that it draws us into our bodies. Our mental electricity twitches through our muscles. We are consumed by our gorgeous internal energy. Still, sometimes that's not always enough to overcome our negative response to the external signs of our aging.

I have a furrow between my brows that can torment me when I look in the mirror. Having become aware of it, I've started to notice when those muscles in my face are engaged. Guess what? Prime time is when I'm pushing myself during a run (or really any workout). Anytime I run hard, I'm deepening the line. I'm not going to stop running. Instead, that furrow has provoked me to think about how to find ease within my effort.

I let my brow be a signpost, reminding me to relax in the midst of my push. To let my body do the work it knows how to do, without force.

October 17

. . . keeping my wrinkles

Chinese medicine says that if we paralyze the muscles of our face and thus our ability to make a certain facial expression (which is what Botox does), then we lose the ability to have the feeling that accompanies that expression. Does that mean that if I can't wrinkle my brow, then I can't run hard? Or that I'll run with more ease, because I can't furrow?

Right now, I'm keeping my wrinkles. While I'm not prepared to say never to cosmetic procedures, for the moment

I'll focus on sleep, water, healthy food, strength, and fulfillment for the ease that smoothes my brow (even if only metaphorically).

October 18

... my inner witch

As I age, the wrinkles on my face tap into my long-held fear that I will become a witch. A woman who, in my imagination, has a fierce, prune face, husky smoker's voice, and an I-can-turn-you-to-stone-with-a-glance demeanor. A type, who when I have encountered her in my life, has always terrified me, because she seemed to possess knowledge about me that even I didn't have access to. The woman who ran the vision quest I went to was such a woman.

The more I try to know myself, the more I feel my inner witch struggling to get out. Some days I even think, *Maybe being a witch isn't so bad.* When they were burned at the stake it was for being independent and strong-minded, for knowing how to cure illnesses with herbs, for hiking around in the woods to collect said herbs, and for being sexually uninhibited.

Independent, wise, vigorous, outdoorsy, and sexy.

I aspire.

October 19

. . . devils wearing Prada

Witches must be distinguished from *Devil Wears Prada* women.

I worked once for such a petty dictator. She had hot and cold running moods, and a fragile belief in her vital role as the final arbiter of literary taste. She propped up her shaky foundation by assigning me menial tasks, utterly unrelated to the job of assistant editor. She often put her dirty winter boots in my inbox for me to messenger home to her apartment. I pulled the rip cord on that job after six long months and found a job featuring mutual respect.

A witch may provoke her sisters, but she never undermines them. Our inner witches are ferocious, sleeping giants, who don't care if they catch more flies with honey, because they don't want flies (who wants flies?). They want truth and justice.

Those brazen hussies. I love them.

October 20

. . . my tiger paws

"Time is the substance I am made of. Time is a river which sweeps me along, but I am the river; it is a tiger which destroys me, but I am the tiger; it is a fire which consumes me, but I am the fire."

—Jorge Luis Borges

I went for a run the morning after I read these words in Borges's 1946 essay, "A New Refutation of Time." As I ran, slower than I had ten years before, I started to think about what I'd carried on my runs the decade past and what I was carrying now. My thoughts became confused. In my memory, events were lining up side by side, when I knew they had been years apart.

"What if *this is all time* right now?" I asked myself. "What if everything I've lived and am going to live is happening right now?"

I felt the river flowing around my feet, the tiger's paws in my shoes. I felt the fire of every run I'd ever done (and maybe those to come) inside my twitching muscles. I ran lighter.

October 21

. . . age-adjusted time

We humans are pretty obsessed by time. Although science and spirituality, in their different but similar ways, often try to tell us that time is not as linear as we think, it's hard for us not to experience it as such. Moving forward. Passing. Slow. Fast.

And when we are athletes, we pile more onto time's back with our pace times, constantly comparing ourselves not only to others but to ourselves the day, the week, the year, the decade before. We act as if time is giving us information more real than any other. We think, *If I used to do 10K in this many minutes and now I do it in this many minutes plus five, then I am verifiably* less. Sure, we can do all the age-adjustment we want, but in our hearts, it is hard not to think, *But I've done better times.*

Remember your tiger's paws!

October 22

. . . meditating on death

In a dharma class I used to go to with a friend, we often did special contemplations on death along the lines, "I could die today." Meditations on death are quite common.

One week when we arrived we learned that the previous week, after our meditation on death, a woman had actually died at the center. My friend and I didn't go back for quite a few months. Our unspoken agreement was to let the karmic-coincidence-level cool down a little.

October 23

. . . snowflake tattoo

Here's a dharma-style story I love:

A dove and a coal mouse are sitting on the branch of a tree, watching the snowfall. The dove asks, "How much does a snowflake weigh?" The coal mouse answers, "Nothing more than nothing." The two birds watch the snowflakes fall for some time more, until the moment a particular one settles on their branch, breaking their perch. As the dove flies away, it thinks to itself, Maybe all that's needed in the world for peace is one more voice.

We can never know if we are the first snowflake, the last snowflake, or any of the snowflakes in between; but we can know that our actions matter. Even if our voice or our actions seem to weigh "nothing more than nothing" in the grand scheme of things—that bottle we recycle, that person we help across the street, or simply the positive energy we radiate—every action is a snowflake, tipping the world toward its better state. If, as Plato believed, the world is because of an ethical need for goodness to exist, then our snowflake behaviors are simply fulfilling our first-principle, cosmic reason to be.

A snowflake tattoo on my left wrist reminds me of this. What I do matters.

October 24

. . . our workouts have purpose

We work out for all sorts of reasons—maybe we do it to de-stress, to get stronger, to be healthy, or for all those ends and others. All good reasons, but beneath this first layer of forces driving us out onto the roads and trails, into the pool, to the yoga studio, or to the gym, resides a sub-layer that is the deeper core of meaning. That is: we nurture our physical, emotional, and spiritual health, so that we can live our best life and fulfill our purpose.

October 25

. . . our health is a resource

"When you make health the goal rather than viewing it as a resource, it's easy to get stressed out, rigid, and narrow-minded. Health is what helps you live the life you want—it's a resource, not a destination."
—Tieraona Low Dog, MD

A physician at the Arizona Center for Integrative Medicine, Low Dog is talking here about the negative stress we can bring to the very act of working out. When our reason to work out is to get thinner, we may beat ourselves up every day that we're not thin enough (never mind by what media-mediated standard we might be judging the result). Or we may work out to get stronger or faster, but in the process actually wear ourselves down, getting weaker and slower (thus cranky, too).

The resource of our good health and wellbeing is a key ingredient in our ability to serve our purpose.

October 26

. . . reclaiming our vitality

Pilar Gerasimo, a journalist and social explorer, takes the idea of health as a resource further still. In her *Manifesto for Thriving in a Mixed-Up World*, she says being healthy is a revolutionary act by which we reclaim our vitality that is both our individual right and our collective responsibility.

Right and responsibility are big words, but that doesn't mean they require big action. Our first responsibility is to the small, everyday things. Most action we take has the power to make the world a better or worse place, including how we treat the people around us. Did you smile at the barista when you got your morning coffee? Or were you scowling for your caffeine, your mind already hours ahead into your day? Bring the energy to your life that you hope for from others.

October 27

. . . lifted in the updraft

How we are in the world matters. How we approach our workouts is just one aspect. You know people who make you feel good, just by being around them. That's who we want to be. And in the end, that's really why we work out.

Sounds heavy. But in fact, adopting this perspective can

bring an incredible lightness to your workouts. Instead of feeling the pressure of the goals you may have set for yourself (that you may be fixating on, or beating yourself up about), you are lifted in the updraft of energy that purpose creates.

October 28

. . . reforestation of the mind

We have dendritic arbors in our brains. Dendrites are the branched projections of a neuron that act to conduct the electrochemical stimulation received from other neural cells to the cell body. As dendrites branch and grow, that branching is called arborization. It's like we have these little forests growing in our brains, the gardens of our mind, without which we can't think, can't act, can't be. The bushier our dendritic arbors, the more able we are to deal with the complexities of the world and, scientists speculate, the happier we are likely to be.

When we lack stimulation, our dendritic arbors begin to wither. As this winter in our brains deepens, our engagement with the world begins to dissolve.

Sports, it turns out, are not just stimulating for our bodies, but our minds, too. When we go out running, or cycling, or dancing, or cross-country skiing, or really whatever moves our bodies vigorously, we can think of it as our personal reforestation program.

Oh, and hugs are important, too (science says so!). I didn't need a study to know that, but it's nice to know there's

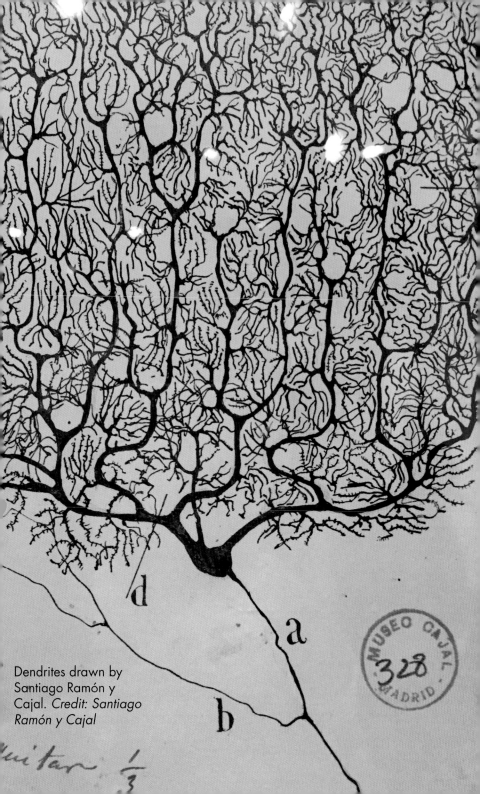

Dendrites drawn by
Santiago Ramón y
Cajal. *Credit: Santiago
Ramón y Cajal*

rigor behind the feeling of wellbeing I have when I hug or am hugged.

So go for a run with a friend tomorrow morning and give her a hug. That's a double bonus-round for bushier dendritic arbors.

October 29

. . . not about the perfect body

As you know by now, I have tried all sorts of different workouts in my time. In addition to all the outdoor sports—running and cycling (off and on road), cross-country skiing, snowshoeing, hiking, kayaking, rock climbing, and swimming— there's yoga (all sorts), barre, spin, aerobics, pole dancing, zumba, kickboxing, indoor rowing, SLT, step classes. I'm sure I've missed something.

Some of these pursuits promise me a perfect body. *I wish*. Actually wait, is that why I'm working out?

Far too many workouts make perfect-body promises. Yet the very idea of perfection is a myth. Do we mean media-generated images of beauty? Because we know that those are manipulated and distorted images of the unreal.

There is no one standard of beauty. The very idea of perfection is a trap, a rat maze with no escape.

To burden our workouts with the end goal of achieving the perfect body is to pursue the impossible dream. Not because you can't do it. Because the end goal does not even exist.

Here's what our workouts should promise us: sweat, a beating heart, better health, and greater pleasure.

October 30

. . . women prefer carrots to sticks

The good news is that deep down we're not so deluded as to be motivated over the long term by the pursuit of the perfect body. Studies show that when we are encouraged in a workout with the carrot of positive reinforcement about the health and happiness benefits of our exercise, then we are far more likely to enjoy and keep doing a workout. Whereas workout environments, which use the stick of negative self-image, shame us into thinking we need a smaller bum, thinner thighs, or a flatter stomach, and so foster recidivism.

Why we work out matters.

The next time you are engaged in your active pursuits, take a mental pause to feel the *why* of your workout. In *Power of Now*, Eckhart Tolle recommends that we scan our physical-emotional being and ask, "Am I happy?"

Lest there's any doubt, we should hope our answer is, "Yes."

October 31

. . . carrots I like

Here are some of the carrots that keep me coming back to my workouts.

I want to be outside—rain, snow, or shine—to feel the elements against my skin and know the seasons are changing by the taste of the air.

I want to be strong, to test my mental and physical endurance, to show myself what I'm capable of.

I want to lounge on my couch in a state of well-earned-body-tiredness with a good book and some chocolate.

I don't want to go gently into that good night, as the poet Dylan Thomas says.

A morning in the mountains: The trail in front of me is streaked with bands of unexplainable light. I blink. I wonder if something is in my eyes. Then I realize that what seems to be coming from inside my eye is actually the sunlight reflected off undisturbed, silk spider filaments, which crisscross my path at ankle level. My heart fills with gratitude for the privilege of such beauty and my luck at being out on the trail. I spread my arms wide and shout nonsense happy-sounds.

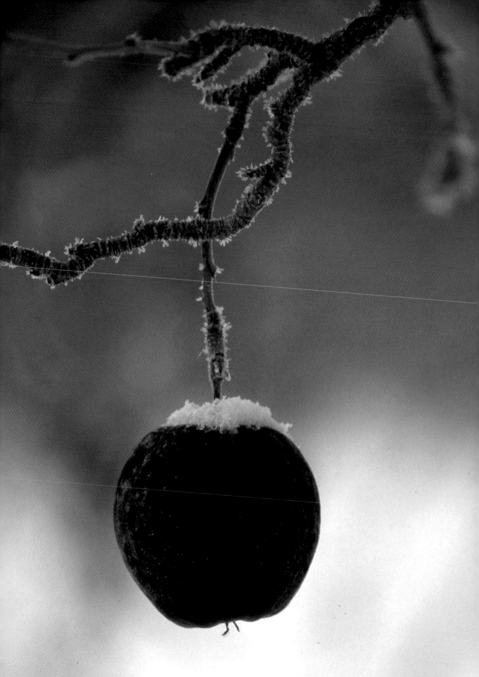

Credit: Joseph Samuels

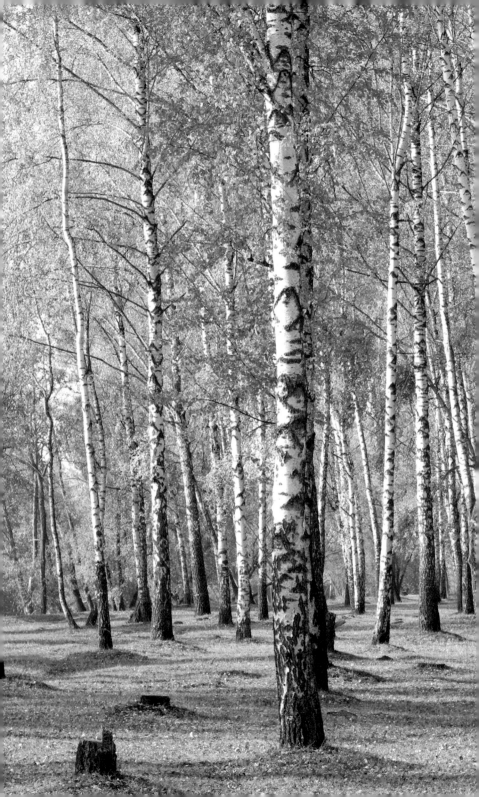

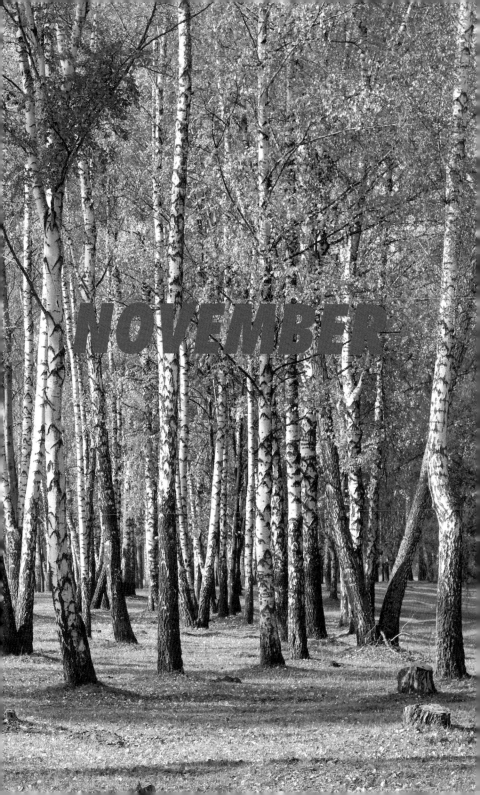

November 1

. . . the dance of compromise and integrity

One of the challenges I wrestle with in life (and in this book) is how we balance our desire to be good people in the world with our basic human need to have fun, to live with joy and lightness. This is what Tamara, the ordained interfaith minister and healer we met earlier, calls "the dance of compromise and integrity."

I will never be, for example, the most perfect environmentalist. I don't know about you, but I'm not prepared to live off the grid. We compromise. At the same time, we try to live in our highest integrity.

November 2

. . . connected to the earth

Tamara is mindful when she surfs. She consciously gives thanks for her close connection with the water and the whole ecosystem it supports. Hiking and running, two other sports she enjoys, feed her connection to the earth.

Our sports are a place to practice our mindful connections with our environment. Whether it's out on a run, or walking to the gym or yoga studio, our natural surroundings deserve our attention and care.

November 3

... forest fires

The forest fires keep getting worse. Where my partner and I live (when we are) in California the smoke rolls in from the fires, blanketing the mountains and hanging over the valleys, filling our lungs. Summer used to be fire season, but now they extend deep into the fall. I haven't even mentioned the droughts, ice caps melting, and A-to-Z storms cycling through the alphabet of names at a furious pace.

The outdoors we play in is demanding our attention, begging for our care.

November 4

... end times

It used to be that only cranks and cult members, people out on the thinnest limbs of sanity, talked about end times. Now the topic is regular cocktail party conversation, global-warming-this, Ebola-that.

Should I be re-thinking my whole life in an attempt to change the course of the world? Or should I just have fun, because the party is almost over?

Enjoy the party, wear your favorite outfit, but clean up throughout the evening. That way, when we wake up in the morning, we can go for our run, knowing we haven't ignored the mess.

November 5

... our holy self is always dancing

The mindful dance we do to find our balance in the world is how we restore and maintain our whole self, our holy self. Our whole self is aware and open, aligned with what is true, authentic and integral to how we are in the world. The closer we are to wholeness, the fewer contradictions exist between our hearts and minds and bodies.

For most of us, there will always be some tension or discord. We are human after all. Acknowledging and reconciling the light and the dark, what Carl Jung called our shadow, is the work of a lifetime (or two or twenty-five). In this lifelong dance, it helps to stop treating our shadow like a villain. Instead, invite it onto the dance floor.

Our holy self is not only willing to dance with our shadow, but also to learn a few new steps.

November 6

... Milarepa

This is a story about Milarepa, the great Tibetan yogi:

One morning Milarepa left his cave to gather firewood. When he returned, his cave was filled with demons. He spent hours, days, weeks, and years trying to chase the demons from his cave. But the more he tried to get rid of them, the more ferocious they became. At last, exhausted from the fight, Milarepa surrendered and invited the demons to stay with him in his cave. Since the demons were so intent on staying, he offered to share his food and shelter. At that moment, all but one of the demons disappeared. The last remaining demon grew to fill the space. Milarepa approached him with humility and put his head in the creature's mouth, now almost as big as the cave itself. There and then the demon dissolved.

In some versions of the story the demons are fire-breathing dragons, but each of us has our own version of the shadows that live inside. I leave their appearance to your imagination.

November 7

. . . a bit of Greek

Our society is very focused on our individuality. We talk about a person's character as their responsibility. This is a view very similar to that of ancient Greek philosophers, as in Aristotle and Plato. There is an ideal of the independent person, a self-starting paragon of discipline.

These Greek ideals of virtue and ethics are excellent. In this book there has been much about our work as individuals to dance with our shadows, forge our paths, be our highest selves.

These are important philosophical and practical ideals. After all, only you can get you out on your morning run.

November 8

. . . a bit of Aztec

Well, actually, a friend can be a big help getting us out on our morning run.

Here's some Aztec philosophy. I didn't know they were a particularly philosophical society, but The Florentine Codex (written by a Spaniard, but so-named because it has been in a library in Florence since the eighteenth century) records their comprehensive systems of thought. For the Aztecs, unlike the Greeks, the focal center of virtue and ethics is found in community, in the support of our family and friends. To lead a worthwhile life, we need the help of other people, plus the additional scaffolding of rituals and routines. In other words, living a good life is a cooperative project, which requires life-long engagement.

Sebastian Purcell writes about this Aztec vision in "Life on the Slippery Earth" for *Aeon*: "Wisdom in human affairs consists in the recognition that the best that we can do is to learn to stand with the help of others, to alter our circumstances for the better, and to clasp hands so that we can pull ourselves back up when we fall."

Reaching for help does not imply weakness or insufficiency. Next time you're relying on a friend for workout motivation, you can think of it as engaging in a bit of Aztec wisdom. And I have no doubt that you will return the support another day.

November 9

. . . The Silkroad Project

The great cellist Yo-Yo Ma founded an organization called The Silkroad Project. Its core mission is to connect across diversity, to bring together musicians from around the globe. Yo-Yo Ma is interested in how people think and express themselves through music, and what they want to communicate with their musical language. These radical cultural collaborations have created surprising and beautiful new music.

Even if we are not musicians, how we live is an expression of our own inner musicality. Our life has a rhythm built on habits and rituals. It has a melody that is our story. We are richer when we reach out across boundaries to understand new ways of doing and being.

November 10

. . . cross training isn't just for our bodies

Greeks. Aztecs. Buddhists. Yo-Yo Ma.

The title of this book may be *Run Like a Girl*, but the running in the title is only a proxy for all the sports we do. And all the sports we do have always been a mirror and microscope on the rest of our lives.

Common sense and our bodies tell us that cross training

will keep us healthier over the long term. Plus—we are more likely to stay engaged with our sports if we mix it up here and there. As much I adore cross-country skiing, I couldn't do it every day. (Well, maybe, if I was faced with one of those improbable desert-island choices.) Cross training works because it engages a wider range of muscles across our whole body. It calls on a spectrum of flexibility, agility, grace, strength, and endurance.

As with our bodies, our brains support each other. There's no one right system of thought. So we seek out new ideas. Test drive. Integrate what resonates and cull what does not. On occasion we should even revisit what we culled and try it on again.

To find the balance, which will afford us our most productive, healthy, and happy life, we must be peripatetic.

November 11

. . . a peach muffin battle

While I was writing about the Greeks and Aztecs and cross training our brains and bodies, I was simultaneously engaged in a mostly silent battle with a peach muffin. Earlier, I'd been seduced by a bakery display. Not the kind of baked treat I'd usually buy. After studying the short, organic ingredients list, I got the peach muffin, full of anticipation.

Back home at my computer, I started writing and eating my muffin. From the first bite, I recognized a food I didn't like enough for the pleasure to outweigh the regret about the wasted calories. Still, I ate through half the muffin. I was hungry for breakfast. Plus I didn't want to waste. After every bite I wrote a little and thought about whether I should stop eating. The muffin and I were in a face off. If I were Aztec, some benevolent person would just take the muffin away from me. My mind got a tangled in what I would do if I were a Greek, a Buddhist, an Aztec, or even Yo-Yo Ma.

Finally, instead of driving myself crazy, I sat for a moment and listened to my body. What did she want? She wanted one of the fresh peaches I'd bought on the same morning excursion.

November 12

. . . growling stomach

My stomach used to growl regularly during meetings back in the days I worked in law firms, but rarely now. I wonder if my stomach was trying to tell me I was in the wrong line of work. I eat better when I'm happier.

November 13

. . . living cubism

Hannah Gadsby, the Australian comic, hates Picasso. She has good reasons, including his homophobia, sexism, and racism. But he did develop a new way of looking at the world through art. Cubism is the simultaneous representation of different points of view—straight on, from above, below, off to the side, from the inside out. In her Netflix special, *Nanette*, Hannah deftly repurposes his artistic style to describe an ideal world: "I want my story heard because ironically, I believe Picasso was right. I believe we could paint a better world, if we learned how to see it from all perspectives, as many perspectives as we possibly could. Because diversity is strength. Difference is a teacher. Fear difference, and you learn nothing."

November 14

. . . eating like a cubist

One day wheat is the devil and the next it's the foundation of an active person's diet. Bananas are either the ultimate quick energy food during an endurance endeavor, or they are the evil cause of belly fat. A new superfood was probably crowned today and will be again tomorrow. Not to mention the crowds of juices and tonics and herbs and spices vying for our attention.

How do we know what to do? Look at the food from as many perspectives as possible and then decide.

Michael Pollan's *Food Rules: An Eater's Manual* lays out three baselines: Eat real food. Not too much. Mostly plants. Real food means not processed, meaning your grandmother could recognize all the ingredients and might have them in her pantry. Here your grandmother and mine and a grandmother from every country in the world are rolled into one uber-global woman with the full breadth of international cuisine knowledge.

I add these things to think about: What is the basis for any health claims? Are the people making the claims the same ones who stand to gain if you buy the food? Are you making rules about what you eat just to feel in control? How does your body feel?

The best for last: pay attention to your food and enjoy, savor, relish!

November 15

. . . superfoods

I love Michael Pollan's counsel for its simplicity and common sense. Yet, I also usually try the latest superfood for its extravagant promises of vampire immortality and dewy skin.

Coco nibs. Goji berries. Jujube fruit. Kombucha. Chia seeds.

Anti-oxidize me. Grant me boundless energy and eternal youth.

If it's an unprocessed food that I can buy without participating in a network-marketing pyramid, I might as well satisfy my curiosity. After all, good food makes us feel good.

November 16

... why I am a vegetarian

There's a Sikh story Tara Brach tells in her book, *Radical Acceptance: Embracing Your Life With the Heart of Buddha*, which conveys why I have been a vegetarian since I was around sixteen years old. The story (summarized from Brach's book):

An ancient wise man summons his two most devout followers. He offers each of them a chicken and says, "Take this chicken where no one can see, and kill it." Without the least hesitation, the first disciple goes behind his hut and cuts off the chicken's head with an ax. The second disciple looks all day and night, finally coming back to his master's doorstep at dawn with the live chicken. When the sage asks him what happened, the disciple says, "There is nowhere I can go that the chicken does not see."

Indeed. I cannot eat a formerly living creature, who I could not look in the eye and then kill. This is a rule for me. So I can look myself in the eye.

November 17

... looking ourselves in the eye

As athletes, we are hyper-keyed into our health. One of the cornerstones of good health—physical, mental, and emotional—is the ability to live comfortably with oneself.

As much thought as we give to our workouts, that and much *more* we need to give to how we are in the world.

November 18

. . . yoga mirror

I don't always want to look myself in the eye. I avoid yoga studios with mirrors. I try to find my yoga alignment from the inside, feeling whether I am correctly aligned. Hands-on adjustments are a big help. But sometimes, there's just going to be a mirror. As much as I'll try not to look, I can't help it.

I am not Gumby. But that hasn't discouraged me from doing yoga for more than twenty years. Some days in yoga I feel strong and aligned and, yes, as if I've captured some of the grace of the practice in my pose. Then I look in the mirror. Is my leg only that high in standing split? Does my upper body not go past 90 degrees in pyramid pose? My leg feels like its reaching for the ceiling. My upper body feels closer to my legs.

Inside, I am doing the poses to my personal highest level of excellence. But the mirror tells me a different story and that can get me a little down. Then a friend talked to me about humility.

November 19

... humble yoga

One day, after a run-in with a yoga mirror, I mentioned the big reality check I'd had to a friend. I told her how I had thought my practice was deepening, and instead I looked like a beginner. Beginner mind is one thing. But, I had beginner body, too. How deflating.

"You're so judgmental," my friend said. "Where's your humility?"

What? Who? Me? Not humble? Wasn't I just being self-critical? Isn't that humble? Not so much.

As my friend wisely pointed out, who was my ego to judge what was excellence in my yoga practice? Did my ego know better than my body what was right and good? Where did my ego get off questioning that little piece of the divine that's in me, in all of us?

Egos aren't good with humility. Who should I trust?—a mirror, or what my body tells me about my effort? I had all the information about the woman I was seeing in the mirror (me!), and still she fell short of my judgment. Imagine how far wrong we can go when we have only the barest sliver of information about other people?

The grace of our practice in anything comes from inside and cannot be judged based on how closely we resemble a photo spread in *Yoga Journal*.

November 20

. . . living without a mirror

I once lived for five months without a full-length mirror. The only mirror where I lived was a small one above the bathroom sink, at head height. I felt so much better about my body during that time than I usually do. When the mirror is there, I look at myself multiple times a day: when I get dressed, maybe to double check before I go out, other times just because I've passed by. Did I look better than usual? Of course not. Why did I go back to living with a full-length mirror? Good question!

November 21

. . . doing math in a bikini

The beauty ideal propagated in our society is ruining girls. Beauty and sexuality have become so completely intertwined as to be indistinguishable. *A Report of the APA Task Force on the Sexualization of Girls* found that the increased sexualization in magazines, marketing, television shows, movies, and song lyrics had the following effects: It harmed girls' interpersonal relationships. It fostered greater body dissatisfaction (as if that issue needs more kindling), and its close companions, eating disorders and increased depression. It generally lessened physical health. And the increased sexualization even led to diminished cognitive skills (apparently the study posed math problems to girls trying on sweaters and girls trying on bathing suits. Those trying on sweaters scored much higher).

The answer is not to stop wearing bikinis or stop doing math. My paternal grandmother was a mathematician at the Bank of Canada in the 1930s. We can and should do both, if that's our jam. It's time to radically rethink beauty.

November 22

. . . mismatched bra and underwear

Wearing a matching bra and underwear is one of my personal foibles. The eccentricity is a hangover from my mother's admonishment to not wear underwear with holes in it, because, what if you got hit by a car? The emergency medics cutting your clothes off to save you would see your hole-y underwear. What kind of impression would that leave?

The underwear doesn't have to be an exact match for the bra, though I do buy *sets* from time to time. But the match has to be very, very close for my satisfaction.

When I dig down into my quirk, I find something more than just a fear of bad drivers. I realize that it makes me feel good in my body to be wearing matching undergarments. It's one of my ways of saying thank you to my body for all the work it does. More—it's a secret superpower that no one knows about except me. Well . . . and now you.

November 23

. . . not just underwear

Yes, though it's not as much of a mania as the bra and underwear business, I do pay close attention to the harmony of my running shoes, socks, skirt, shirt, and hat (if it's sunny). I just feel better when my clothes aren't arguing with each other. I know I'm not alone in this. An informal Facebook survey I did showed that a significant majority of women coordinate their sweat couture. The breakdown is about even between women who match what's underneath.

November 24

. . . getting kicked out of gym class

When I was around fifteen, I got kicked out of gym class for wearing shorts and a t-shirt that didn't match. Not wearing the gym uniform would have been forgivable, or so my gym teacher told me, as she escorted me from the gym. But apparently I had chosen to wear a t-shirt that clashed so appallingly—a bright red shirt worn with the purple uniform shorts—that the teacher couldn't even tolerate me in class. At the time I was pretty proud of myself for that fashion criminality, because I didn't like gym class to begin with. I took some pleasure in annoying my teacher, who didn't bother to hide the fact that she didn't think much of my athletic abilities. Just for the record, I was fleet-ish as a kid, but would have required some encouragement.

I sometimes fantasize about an athletic competition with that gym teacher—me, at my current age and ability; and her, at her then-age and ability. I'll wear whatever uniform she deems appropriate.

November 25

. . . first-world problem

Yes, fashion is a first-world problem. If we want to be hard on ourselves, we could judge our concern with color coordination as frivolous in a world where people don't have enough to eat, but then again, the first world is where I (and likely, you) live. Pretty much all of our problems will be of that world. To apply a blanket discount to the things that concern us day-to-day is to discount our existence.

To bowdlerize Descartes (especially now that we know we are Merlau-Pontians), I exist, therefore I will continue to make an effort to match. That doesn't stop us from thinking about how we contribute to making the world a better place, but these few days here are about clothing and how it makes us feel.

November 26

. . . six reasons to match

Without further ado, based on my oh-so-scientific research and a little look inside my own head, here are six reasons to match:

1. You match your non-workout clothes. Why not match what you work out in? What you wear makes a statement, no matter the activity in which you are engaged.
2. When you look good, you feel good. We all know that more than half the battle in a workout (in life, really) is our mental condition. Why not give your self-image the best environment you can create.
3. An outfit you love may be the difference between getting out for a workout or not.
4. When you look good, you inspire others to make the same effort, which repays them in all the ways already mentioned.
5. On top of which, a super-fly outfit might just give you the edge you need on the other competitors. (Serena Williams shows us how!)
6. Last but not least, take the outward appearance to another level deeper, if you don't already. Matching bra and underwear are a secret superpower. Try it!

November 27

. . . like an OzGoth

I once went to a burlesque/cabaret/aerial/magic show. The performers were . . . mostly great. The MC of the evening had that disconcerting "pick-on-people" manner. He singled me out to make fun of my style as some combination of Goth and Wizard of Oz. For the rest of the evening he referred to me as OzGoth.

I was pretty crushed. In the moment, I did that gamely-girl thing of smiling, as if I didn't care that he'd just told me he thought I looked weird. To be fair, he was meaner to other people. But still, it hurt. I had been feeling pretty good about myself the moment before. I'd had a great cross-country ski that morning. I was wearing a new outfit that made me feel groovy. I was with my partner and close friends. And just like that, *pop!* went my balloon of wellbeing. Even the next day I felt bad about what the MC had said to me.

After a few days I started to see things differently. I started to think—what is OzGoth, really?—A combination of the rebellion of Goth with the sparkly optimism of The Wizard of Oz; which makes me an optimistic rebel. Sold!

Is this an idea for a new line of running gear?

November 28

. . . are running shoes shoes or gear?

While I've been working on this book, I've also been engaged with my annual challenge. For the past few years I've tried to do something new or different every year—fast one day a month, end every shower with cold water. This year my goal is not shopping for clothes, shoes, handbags, or jewelry.

It's a challenge to be sure. Also, detoxifying. And I will look forward to some new clothes come January.

One of the questions people keep asking me is, "What about running shoes?"

This is my answer: Running shoes are gear. They keep my body safe from injury. And . . . there is a "but." I have two pairs that were relatively fresh on January 1 and I cross train. I think I can make it without buying a new pair.

In case you're interested, I did the math. Fifty-two weeks in the year. Twelve weeks in California, either cross-country skiing in the winter or trail running in the summer (so not using my road running shoes) = forty weeks maximum of road running. At the most I run thirty road miles a week now (trails are a different story). Twelve hundred miles ÷ two = six hundred miles/per pair. That's pushing it, but not extreme. Hello fresh insoles.

If I feel even a twinge, I'll buy new shoes.

November 29

. . . what if this is the best day?

Every once in a while I have a day where I feel like the universe has noticed me. On one such day, Wednesday, November 29, 2017, to be precise, I was riding Citibike down to yoga. It was the middle of the day. A gorgeous day. Cool and crisp. Blue sky. Grey ripple of the river to my right. My partner and I had gotten into a bit of a *discussion* in the morning over breakfast, which we had managed to resolve quite amicably. A new skill for us. I had been writing in the morning, working on a particular project that I was into quite deeply. Now it was lunch hour and I had the luck to be outside in the fresh air, headed to a class with one of my favorite instructors.

For some reason I had this thought: What if this is the best day of all the days there are to come in my life? I was cycling past new concrete barriers designed to stop another terrorist driving a truck down the bike path. Giant icebergs were calving off glaciers, which hold back waters that can raise the sea level. My thought ballooned. I took stock of everything I was grateful for in my life—my partner, my health, my work, my cat, my family, my friends, the river, the trees, the earth, and more. Until my heart could hardly hold the thought it grew so big.

I was filled with joy.

November 30

. . . Because I Am Your Queen

My thought continued: What if you never publish another book? What if your fable translations come to nothing? What if your play never sees a stage light?

I was still filled with joy.

I was joyful all through my class.

On the elevator after class, I pulled out my cell phone. I thought, *Why can't you just not look at your device until you get home?* I looked. There was an email from a professor at a theatre department. A play I'd created with three other collaborators was being considered for their program. I thought, *I am so happy right now that I can take this news. Then I can ride off the rejection sadness on the way home.*

The department had chosen my new play *Because I Am Your Queen* for a March 2019 production. Remember that high kick of ninja-confidence back in March? It was for this play. Never mind that the success came through another door.

I started crying on the street.

Any number of philosophies counsels us to let go, that the universe will do its work; that our happiness is in our hands (or really our minds), regardless of circumstance. I know it's true. Intellectually. But I sure have a hard time actually executing it.

I didn't try to let go. It just happened. I'm not sure I know how to let go again. But now I know the feeling. I can practice.

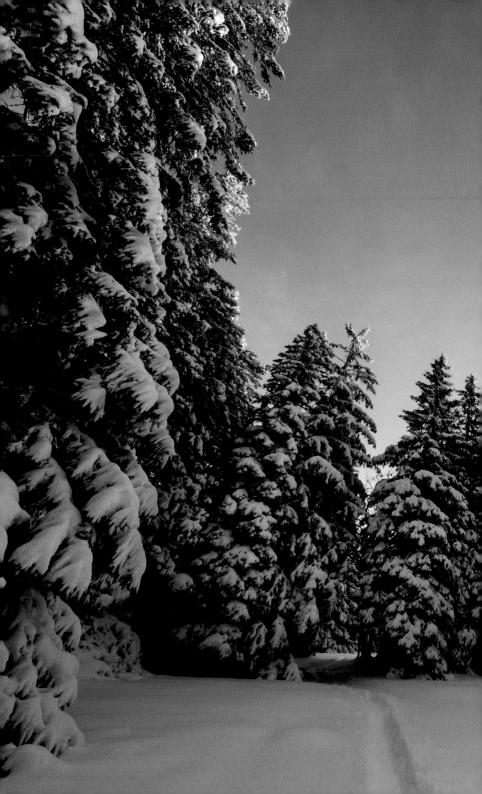

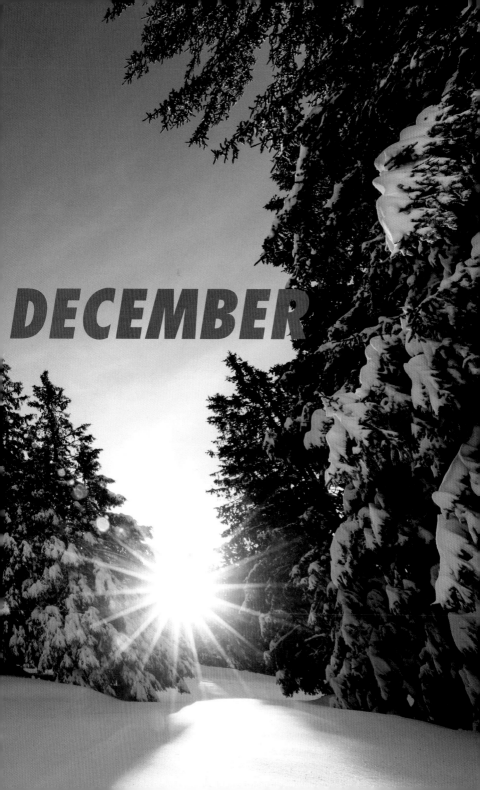

DECEMBER

December 1

. . . time

As we begin the last month of the year, time is on my mind. The way time bends and loops. The way time compresses in a moment of such profound happiness that we almost feel its density, like the day I described on November 29. How time stretches endlessly around a *when-will-this-be-over* moment, like the midsection of a long race.

My tiger's paws are tingling in Borges's river and fire.

December 2

. . . clueless

I do yoga and meditate. I've gone to silent retreats. I've done a vision quest, fasting alone in the desert. The whole shebang. Yet, most days I feel like I haven't got a clue about anything.

Maybe that's the point.

December 3

. . . the little things

I once had bronchitis. My coughing was severe enough that I fractured ribs on both sides. I had never spent so many weeks in bed. Before the bronchitis, I had never even broken a bone. The weeks of bronchitis were unlike anything I'd experienced before.

During that time, I stepped out of the current of my own life. The world was moving on around me, but I slowed to a near stop. Week by week, I cancelled everything on my calendar. A shortlist of things I couldn't do: breathing, eating, drinking, getting into or out of bed, putting on underwear, spitting out toothpaste, opening the heavy front door of my apartment building, laughing. Almost daily I re-jigged my expectations of myself. Once I was out of bed, I started walking in the morning at quarter speed. When a fleet woman glided by, legs roped with working muscles, I'd want to cry.

But there was also pleasure in the new pace. I noticed the little things. One day, as I caught up to a man walking even more slowly than I was, I smelled his baby before I saw the infant in his arms, that sour-milk-powdery-sleep scent of the first months of life. Running, I would never have caught that whiff, I would have passed by too quickly.

December 4

. . . stillness and gusto

While I was laid up, I read a Buddhist blog, which encouraged, in typical Buddhist fashion, slowing down, savoring, for example, each small sip of a glass of water—something I was forced into by my bronchitis.

While stillness is a practice worth cultivating, I love gulping down my water with gusto. To get to the end of a long, hot workout and pour something cool down my throat—what a superb privilege. Noticing the small pleasures does not always require that they be slow and measured. Noticing matters more than the stillness.

In low moments when I was sick, I longed to sink beneath the waters of self-pity. I wondered if I'd ever get better. I wondered who I was. I wanted an explanation of why I was sick.

I like to think of myself as having a high pain tolerance. Before I knew my ribs were fractured, I was self-critical about the amount of pain I was feeling. Then I thought I should be able to get through the rib pain without depending on the prescribed painkillers. I kept reassessing and finding myself falling short. I wanted to hang onto some preconceived notion of strength and resilience with which I identified myself. As if I might lose the self I thought I was.

Buddhism counsels us to shed our ego, the self I was fighting hard to hang onto. When we are well, it feels easy to contemplate the no-self. How much harder it is when we are sick.

December 5

... show up like you mean it

You may have noticed that I think a lot about an eternally provocative question: *Why are we here?* Maybe there doesn't need to be an answer. But isn't it nice to have a reason to show up for something as important as our existence? At a fundamental level, think of how much more reliable and motivated you are when someone else is counting on you. Showing up feels good. Think how much you appreciate your workout partners. We need to show up for our lives and the world. Our presence is important.

December 6

... want to do more

I was reminded of the importance of showing up in a stark way while reading Leymah Gbowee's *Mighty Be Our Powers.* The book is about Leymah coming into her womanhood and finding her strength and activist core in Liberia during the brutal civil war.

Writing about coming out of a long depression (brought on by an abusive relationship, not to mention the horrors of the violence in Liberia), Leymah begins to feel the power of meaning in her life: "I wasn't sitting home thinking endlessly about what a failure I was; I was doing something, something that actually helped people. The more I did, the more I could do, the more I wanted to do, the more I saw needed to be done."

Most of us are lucky enough not to face such overwhelming challenges. Our worlds are relatively peaceful and easy. Complacence is natural. Still, most of us have days we hide away, feeling like failures, until something demands our presence and there's no space left for despondency. What we show up for can start as simple as a run.

December 7

. . . beyond a bake sale

Paloma started running in the seventh grade, when one of her friends encouraged her to join the cross-country team. The distances seemed crazy long at first, but it didn't take much time before Paloma fell in love with the running off-road. When her small team of five girls got to high school, they decided they at least needed t-shirts for competitions. Paloma, passing over the traditional bake sale route, suggested the team organize a 5K event in town for girls and women only, as a way of fundraising for their team. One hundred and fifty women turned out the first year.

"I realized this was about more than raising money for my cross-country team," Paloma says. "I saw how invigorating and powerful and supportive it was to have a women-only event. And hearing the women's stories, 'this is my first 5K' or 'this is my first run since my husband's death,' it was amazing to feel that I was helping women through things in their lives, and helping them feel active, healthy and productive."

That same year, Paloma founded the organization Simply Women Ohio. In addition to hosting the annual 5K, Simply Women has a mission to blaze a trail for women athletes in Yellow Springs, Ohio.

Not all of us find our purpose as early in life as Paloma, and that's perfectly fine. Start simple. Start when the time is right for you.

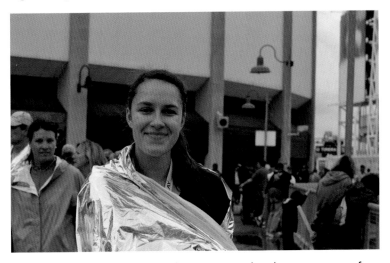

Caption: Paloma at the end of a race. *Credit: Photo courtesy of Paloma*

December 8

. . . flow for humankind

We each have our own personal missions of strength and endurance. Such quests, as Mihaly Csikszentmihalyi wrote in his classic book *Flow*, enable us to expand our concepts of ourselves, which, in turn, builds the self-confidence that "allows us to develop skills and make significant contributions to humankind."

Yes!

December 9

. . . celebrating without mascara

When Czech snowboarder Ester Ledecká won the women's super-G at the 2018 Winter Olympics, no one was more shocked than she. After all, she'd borrowed a pair of skis for the event. Why? Because she was a snowboarder. No surprise, the press mobbed her for interviews immediately after her gold medal run, during which she never took off her ski goggles. Weird. Did she just forget?

Nope. It was because she wasn't wearing mascara, since she had absolutely no expectation of even placing in the event. Apparently, all the other women who thought they had a chance of being on the podium wore mascara, just in case. I didn't even know that was a thing.

I got a little steamed. Seriously? A woman wins a gold medal, but the pressure to look pretty and perfect is so strong that she doesn't want to be seen without mascara after her victory. This is a woman who has just completed a gorgeous athletic feat.

What more does society want from women?

December 10

... confession about my eyelashes and eyebrows

I need to confess that although I never wear makeup when I'm working out and barely ever wear it otherwise, I do in fact tint my invisible eyelashes. I also have an eyeliner and eyebrow tattoo, to cut down on more tinting maintenance responsibilities.

Am I a hypocrite about Ester Ledecka? Is my feminism suspect? I could make all sorts of excuses about my age and her youth. Each of us has different standards. Very few of us are pure and consistent 100 percent of the time.

I'm sad that winning at the Olympics is not always enough for a woman to feel beautiful in that moment.

December 11

... no rose

The first marathon I did, I was so far off the goal I'd set that I started crying after the finish line. I refused to take the finisher's medal or the red rose (thorns removed). It's a good thing I wasn't wearing mascara. It would have run.

December 12

. . . on balance

When my father was dying he made a point of having some last conversations. He was always organized that way.

He told me that when his mother (my grandma) died, she told him I was unhappy. She wasn't wrong. I was twenty-two, in the wrong relationship, and headed down the wrong career path. My self-esteem was in the garbage can. But you know all that already.

My father saw me in a different light. "Why weren't you happy?" he asked me. "You were always so good at everything you set your mind to."

Was I? Am I? No. Yes. A bit of both.

I know this: I'm happy now. Not every minute. But a lot of minutes. It's a balance.

I told him that, so he could rest easy. And maybe he's let my grandmother know, if he sees her where he is.

December 13

. . . cross-country skiing with my father

I don't have any particular memories of cross-country skiing with my father, but I know I did as a child. There are pictures to prove it. I stopped cross-country skiing in my teens and didn't start again until my mid-thirties. I never cross-country skied with my father as an adult. That is, until after he died.

Climbing out of the Euer Valley the winter after his death, my heart punching against my chest like a prisoner in despair, I felt my lips contract into the shape of an O. I heard the bubbly intake of saliva through my teeth in the exact way my father used to do, when he was pushing against a wall of effort. It was the same breath he took when he was beginning to relish a debate. I could recognize his signature intake of concentrated breath with my eyes closed. It found me cross-country skiing.

In the same moment I became aware of thoughts that weren't mine. They were in his voice, "I can do this. Hang on a second. I almost have it. If I can just . . ."

No sooner was I aware of his presence as I skied, than he was gone. I was me again, skiing uphill, exhausted. Sad. Also happy.

December 14

. . . angel dust

He skied with me one other time. An early morning, my partner and I were the first tracks on the fresh white corduroy; the only sound the *swish-whisper-scrape* of our skis across the snow, grainy with cold. At first I thought I was hearing someone skiing up on me from behind, but there was no one. After I'd looked around for the third time I realized it was my father who I was feeling.

I was with him when he died, a stroke of luck, as strange

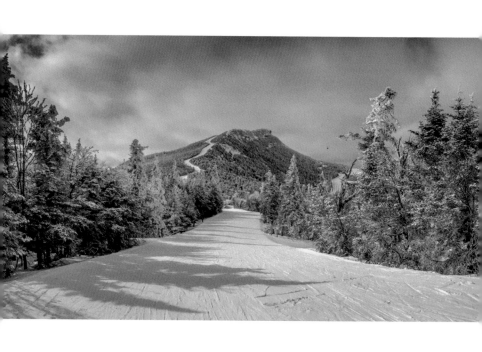

as that may sound. But it granted me the privilege of feeling the sizzle of energy as his solid-earth life left him, and that electric sparkle of angel dust passed through space, through me, assuring me that he wasn't gone. He was transformed, a radiance in the universe that I might feel from time to time, if I was willing. And yet, he was also gone, an understanding that has sunk in slowly, every time I think of him, and realize, as if anew, his physical absence.

December 15

. . . the elixir

"It is death that consoles, alas, and makes us live;/ It is the goal of life, and its only hope/ that, like an elixir, elevates us and intoxicates us/ And gives us the heart to walk into the night;/ Through the storm, and the snow and the frost/ It is the terrace that opens on the unknown skies!"

That's French poet Charles Baudelaire's "The Death of the Poor" (my translation).

I can't choose when my father's energy will manifest from those unknown skies, but I am consoled, elevated and, yes, even intoxicated, by the knowledge that death is more mysterious than I expected. I hope he'll ski with me again.

December 16

...pictures for my father

Flying into Boise, Idaho for the first time, the rolling desert—brown, arid, sensual—surprised me. I often imagine walking into that kind of terrain and never returning. *Snap*.

The sky is twilight orange, streaked with clouds curving into the horizon, smudged by a thin veil of forest fire smoke. *Snap*.

I was snapping mental pictures for my father. Five months after my father died, he was more present to me than he had been since my childhood.

I started sending the photos to him when I was on a trip to Colorado, shortly before my father was diagnosed with melanoma. He liked getting the snapshots. I kept on, sending him glimpses of what I saw—a man's hat on the subway (shot from the hip), railway girders swooshing by against a night sky from a train window, an unexpected herd of sheep on a mountain bike ride.

Once my father told me that I had a good eye. I stowed that compliment away in my pocket, like a lucky pebble, shining his words between my thumb and forefinger when I was thinking of him. It was the most regular contact I'd had with him for years.

Snap. I took a picture of a sunflower while running on the Camelback trails in Boise. It was for my father.

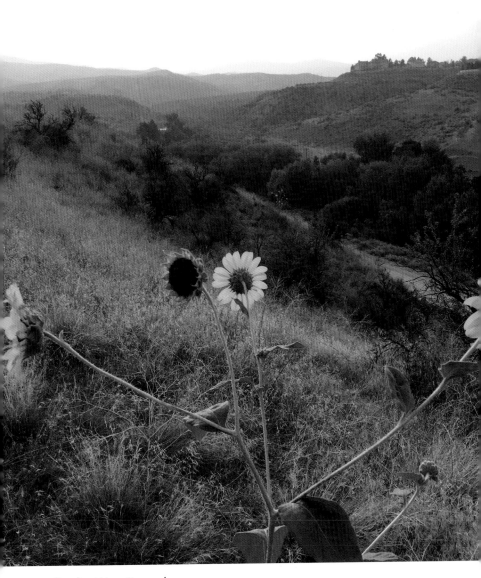

Credit: Mina Samuels

December 17

. . . afternoon naps

Some people think naps are the enemy of drive and ambition. Not me. An afternoon nap is a gift (my father loved them even more). I have trouble feeling ambitious when I'm exhausted. Also, on Saturday afternoons, after a long weekend workout, even if I'm not particularly tired, the delicious, decadence of a little lie-down takes precedence over the future of my life.

December 18

. . . the fine line

We like to think that our athletics are all to our benefit. After all, our sports give us vitality and strength. They teach us about self-motivation, hard work, setting and meeting goals. Being athletic can make us more conscious of how we fuel our bodies. Tamara's sports led her into healthier eating habits, which healed a digestive disorder and leaky gut from eating too much processed food.

Yet, as Tamara points out, celebrating our strength as beauty is empowering, until it tips over into an excessive focus on our bodies. When we push girls into a hyper-competitive mindset, we may negate the feminine gifts of intuition and nurturance. There is a fine line between the benefits and the perils. Tamara knows. As an ordained interfaith minister and healer, she sits in council circles with girls struggling to find their place in the world.

Our effort, as always, is to find the balance; so that our sports support our bodies and our lives in a holistic way.

December 19

. . . straightening out the wires

It's been ten years since Paloma founded Simply Women Ohio to support her high school cross-country team. Since then, she's graduated from Smith College and is exploring work and training in the fields of health and healthcare access, incorporating holistic medicine in her skill set.

Her relationship with running has been complicated these last years. She tore her Achilles in her last year of high school and couldn't run for two years. Then, just as she was getting back into running, she tore a calf muscle, and had to get surgery. She switched to other sports—power lifting, swimming, and biking. None are the same. Paloma says running is the one thing that, "Gets the wires straightened out and helps me sort things out."

She was angry about not running during a lot of college. "I'm not sure I recalibrated as successfully as I could have." She wonders if she might have taken more pride in her academic work, if she'd had running as a pick-me-up, to refocus, and to study and sleep better.

Now she's consciously finding other productive and healthy coping mechanisms—other sports, new fields of study—so that she has the balance to find her sense of wellbeing not just in running, but from multiple sources. She knows, too, that really there is just the one ultimate source, and that's her own sense of self-efficacy and strength. She's a wise young woman.

December 20

. . . raw self-love

In an interview with *Trail Runner* magazine after the Western States (that's a one-hundred-mile trail-run event) in 2018, Lucy Bartholomew, an Australian ultra-runner, described her relationship to running as "the most powerful and raw form of self care and self love."

How thrilling and fortunate, when we can find these things inside ourselves.

December 21

. . . ping-pong

A few years ago my partner and I got a ping-pong table. We play in our garage in Truckee. And when we're not playing the table folds up and rolls into the corner. Even when I'm grumpy because I'm losing, it's a fun way to unwind at the end of a workday. The game has been a steep learning curve, because I never played until a few years ago. I've discovered that if I work on catching the ping-pong ball with my left hand (another element of my ambidexterity project), then I play better, even though I hold the paddle with my right. In the winter catching the ball requires extra skill, because I'm wearing fingerless gloves, because unheated garage and winter.

December 22

. . . integrationism

I learned recently that on many days I'm an integrationist when it comes to physical activity.

Integrationists are people who, yes, workout, but the crux of the definition is they are also physically active throughout their day. Taking stairs instead of elevators. Riding a bike to commute. Walking. In other words, people who integrate movement into their lives, whether or not they're formally working out. Their opposites are called compartmentalists. Their workouts may be as hard as they come, but then they don't move the rest of their day.

I thought I was just unwinding at the end of the day with a bit of ping-pong. I loved finding out there was a formal word to describe what I was intuitively doing—integrationism.

December 23

. . . integrate

I like the word, in all its forms. Integration implies balance and harmony. Integrating movement in our days. Integrating our public selves and private selves to be more authentic. Integrating our emotions, instead of pretending we can compartmentalize and ignore them. Integrating work and pleasure, so that the former is not something we dread.

It's lovely.

December 24

. . . the real challenge

Integration. Balance. Happiness. Fulfillment. Meaning. Purpose. Everywhere we turn now, from workout class instructors to apps, to this book, we are bombarded with quotes and encouragements that are meant to inspire us. Are the words standing in for the actual need to be mindful? Are we all dispensing and receiving aphorisms like tiny candies? Are we robbing them of their essential truth? Have we been lulled into thinking that somehow just hearing the words is all that's required of us?

The real challenge facing each of us is this—how can we elevate the barrage of mindfulness blandishments into true, heightened, self-awareness and real, effective action to make the world a better place?

December 25

. . . the good side

One of the very simple, central tenets of Zoroastrianism (possibly the most ancient organized religion) is this: Knowing the world is made up of good and evil, the Zoroastrian asks herself every morning, "Which side am I on?"

Every day is an opportunity to have good thoughts, speak good words and take good actions; in other words, an opportunity to reclaim our vitality.

December 26

. . . power over ourselves

"I do not wish them [women] to have power over men; but over themselves."

So wrote Mary Wollstonecraft in *A Vindication of the Rights of Woman.*

Sports give us power over ourselves. Let's exercise that power well.

December 27

...like a girl

Fast and furious.
   Powerful and strong.

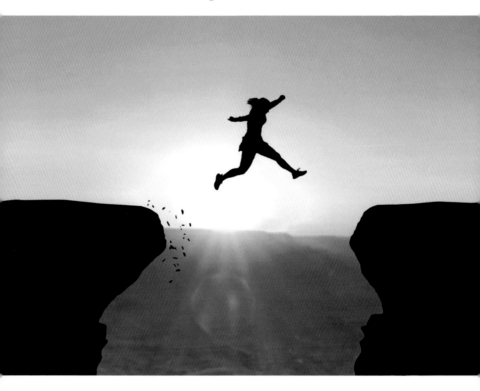

December 28

. . . like a girl

Kicking some butt.
Running hard and winning.

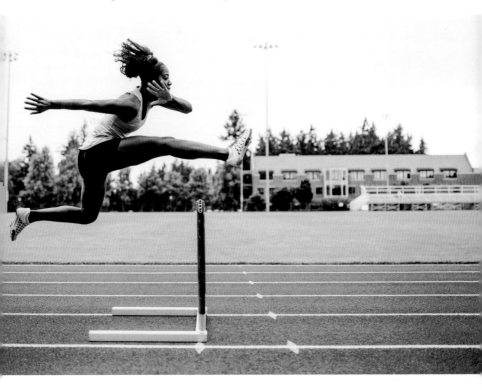

December 29

. . . like a girl

Delighted and exuberant.
Dreamy and unselfconscious.

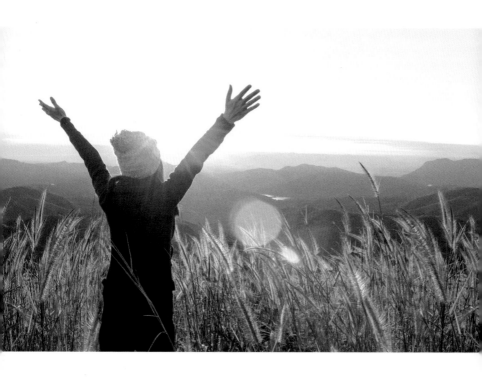

December 30

. . . like a girl

Plunging forward into life.
Playing.

December 31

. . . like a woman

Let's carry those girl qualities into the women we are, so that we can be our own full authentic selves, finding and giving joy.

Run like a girl. Be a strong woman. Let your life speak for all of us to hear.

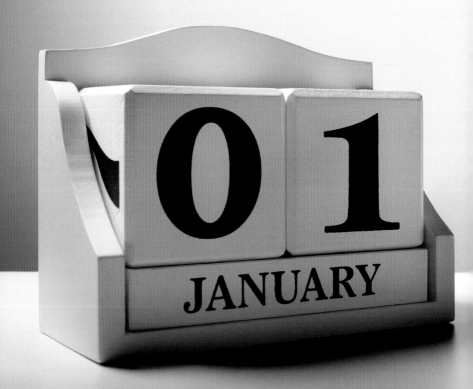

JANUARY

. . . ready, set, GO!

January 1

. . . a word

New beginning. Fresh start.
We're here again.
What's your word?
Mine is FLUID.

ACKNOWLEDGMENTS

The women who so generously shared their stories— you are always an inspiration to me. The women I've shared the roads and trails with—you continue to show me how to run like a girl. My keen readers along the way— Rachel Makofsky, Sherrye Henry Jr., Ronnie Alvarado, my editor, and Lisa Leshne, my agent. Always and above all, David Foster, my most generous reader, supporter, partner and true companion.

ABOUT THE AUTHOR

Mina Samuels is a writer, performer, athlete, citizen, and enthusiast. Her previous books include *Run Like a Girl: How Strong Women Make Happy Lives*, *The Queen of Cups*, and *The Think Big Manifesto*, co-authored with Michael Port. She has written and performed two one-woman plays: *Do You Know Me?* and *Hazards*, as well as written an ensemble play, *Because I Am Your Queen*. She lives in New York City and Truckee, California.

NOTES

_____

_____

_____

_____

_____

_____

_____

_____

_____

_____